Y0-BCL-300

SCIENCE PRINCIPLES APPLIED TO NURSING

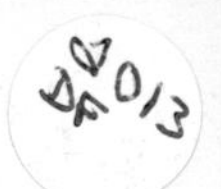

SCIENCE PRINCIPLES APPLIED TO NURSING:

A REFERENCE FOR NURSE EDUCATORS

MADELYN TITUS NORDMARK, R.N., B.S., M.S. (N.E.)
Research Assistant Professor, School of Nursing
University of Washington

ANNE W. ROHWEDER, R.N., B.S., M.N.
Research Assistant Professor, School of Nursing
University of Washington

Foreword by MARY S. TSCHUDIN
Dean, School of Nursing, University of Washington

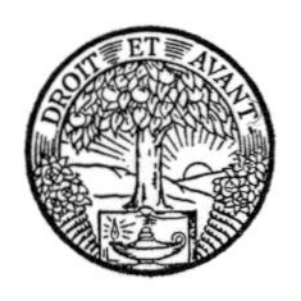

J. B. LIPPINCOTT COMPANY
Philadelphia and Montreal

Second Printing

Distributed in Great Britain by
Pitman Medical Publishing Co., Limited, London

Library of Congress Catalog Card No. 59-10543

Printed in the United States of America

Contents

FOREWORD

THE importance of the social, physical and biological sciences in nursing education has been emphasized repeatedly. The student is expected to draw upon all the science knowledge she possesses and to apply this knowledge in a variety of nursing situations. She is expected to see the relationships between many facts, principles and concepts and their relevance to particular problems in nursing; and, from this background, to make sound decisions for her nursing actions.

With the rapid expansion of scientific knowledge relevant to nursing care, the task of helping the student to achieve this level of performance becomes a major challenge for nursing educators. There is need to promote continued learning of the sciences throughout the educational program and to extend the meaningfulness of this knowledge for effective patient care.

This book presents the results of an extensive study of the application of social and natural science principles in nursing which was conducted at the University of Washington. A major portion of the material, which has been organized to facilitate its use by teachers, is devoted to the presentation of principles from psychology, sociology and anthropology, and from chemistry, physics, anatomy, physiology and microbiology, all of which are important to nursing. Accompanying each group of principles are the related statements of nursing care. Suggestions are offered to show how students may be helped to develop a greater understanding of the relevance of science to effective nursing care.

It is hoped that as teachers use the materials presented in this book, they will be stimulated to identify additional principles from the social and natural sciences and their implications for nursing practice.

Mary S. Tschudin, Dean
School of Nursing
University of Washington
Seattle, Washington

ACKNOWLEDGEMENTS

For many years nurse educators have shown a growing appreciation of the contributions of the basic sciences to nursing. This appreciation has led to the recognition of the need to delineate specifically the application of sciences to nursing practice. In addition, there has been an intensification of the felt need in the nursing profession for the formulation of a fundamental core of nursing knowledge. These two needs stimulated the study which is reported in this publication—an investigation which was supported by The Commonwealth Fund and carried out in the University of Washington School of Nursing.

A study of this kind cannot be accomplished without the cooperation and sustained efforts of many people. The authors wish to acknowledge, first of all, the members of the Natural and Social Science Committees of the University of Washington School of Nursing who faithfully gave their time and energies during the five-year period. Members of the Natural Science Committee included: Helen Anderson, Helen Belcher, Lucy Enos, Shirley Fredrickson, Julie Hanson, Stella Hay, Priscilla Normark, Bessie Robinson and Vesta Franz Skeins. Members of the Social Science Committee included: Viola Brown, Dorothy Burke, Marguerite Cobb, Betty Jane Ely, Betty Hart, Edith Heineman, Charity Kerby, Dolores Little, Mary O'Brien, Betty Olsen Ames, Maxine Patrick, Eleanor Perdelwitz, Lorraine Phillips, Patricia Rose, Patricia VanderLeest, Harriet Ulrich and Frances Zaleski.

The task of identifying important principles from the natural sciences was greatly aided by the major contributions of several of the teachers of science at the University of Washington. Dr. Julia Skahen, Assistant Professor of Physiology, Biophysics and Anatomy, devoted innumerable hours of her time to the study.

Also of great assistance were Dr. B. S. Henry, Professor of Microbiology, Dr. S. G. Powell, Professor of Chemistry, and Dr. L. A. Sanderman, Associate Professor of Physics.

The following medical specialists were most gracious and helpful in reviewing and criticizing the nursing care principles related to the natural sciences; Doctors Robert M. Paine, Fred Casserd, Alexander P. Greer, Louis N. Hungerford, Jr., Hugh Jones, John F. Le Cocq, Edward H. Morgan, Gerald Nowlis, Robert Pommerening, William J. Steenrod, Jr. and Heston L. Wilson.

For the collection of data for the social science portion of the study, the efforts of the nursing personnel in the five participating hospitals are particulary appreciated: King County Hospital, Northern State Hospital, Swedish Hospital, Seattle Veterans' Administration Hospital and Virginia Mason Hospital.

Special thanks go to Doctors Ivar Lovaas and James Taylor of the University of Washington Department of Psychology for reviewing and criticizing the social science data.

The authors are grateful to the members of both juries who evaluated the total data.

Much of the study was more easily facilitated by the secretarial assistance of Miss Doris Kelly, Mrs. Lois Martin and Mrs. Carolyn Miller.

The support and encouragements which the authors received from the entire faculty of the University of Washington School of Nursing was invaluable. Last, but by no means least, special thanks go to Dean Mary S. Tschudin and Assistant Dean Katherine Hoffman for their consistent support.

Anne W. Rohweder
Madelyn T. Nordmark
Seattle, Washington
December 25, 1958

Part One

CHAPTER I: *Orientation*

INTRODUCTION

THE nurse is constantly called upon to make independent decisions in the solution of such problems as those concerned with patient care, safety for herself and others, and interpersonal relationships. Increasingly, she is expected not only to make wise decisions for herself but to guide auxiliary personnel who perform nursing care functions. In the process of executing nursing activities the nurse cannot always find a policy, a "rule of thumb", or a person of authority to assist her when a problem arises. Even if comprehensive sets of rules were available, the habitual use of such rules would be potentially dangerous in that they could very likely lead to unthinking and harmful actions because the nurse failed to understand the reasons behind the behavior. It would seem vital, then, that the professional nurse be equipped to solve problems in a wise and resourceful manner.

The successful use of problem-solving methods—which, hopefully, the nurse will employ in making her decisions—implies that the problem-solver has in her possession, or at her disposal, the facts and understandings necessary for the analysis and solution of problems. This implication leads to two significant questions for nurse educators:

> What facts and understandings are important for a professional nurse to have in her possession?
> How can these facts and understandings and their use in solving nursing problems be learned most effectively?

Recognition of the significance of these questions led the original planners of the five-year curriculum study in basic nursing education at the University of Washington School of Nursing[1] to select the relating of the general and professional education of nursing students as one area for investigation.

The Commonwealth Fund first supported this separate study, within the framework of the total curriculum study, for a three-year period. During this time two investigators studied several aspects of the over-all problem. The specific problems isolated for study were:

1. Which principles from the basic sciences does a professional nurse need to know?
2. How can students best be helped to develop the ability to apply these principles to the solution of problems in nursing care?
3. How can student growth toward the achievement of this ability be evaluated?
4. How can the regular clinical faculty be helped to increase their ability to integrate social and natural sciences into the teaching program?

Although all four of the above problem areas were studied to some extent, time limitations and other requirements of the total curriculum study necessitated the placing of emphasis upon the study of teaching and evaluation methods.[2] As the study progressed, the need to determine specific basic science facts and understandings applicable to nursing became increasingly obvious. This problem was given consideration to some extent, but it was apparent that any real contribution in this area would demand concentrated study over a period of time. For this reason, near the close of the original three-year study the Commonwealth Fund was asked to extend support for an

[1] Sand, Ole: Curriculum Study in Basic Nursing Education, 225 pp., New York, Putnam, 1955.

[2] Rohweder, Anne W. and Titus, Madelyn: A Study of the Application of Basic Sciences to Nursing: A Cumulative Report Covering the Period from December, 1953 to December, 1956. 92 pp., Univ. Washington Press, 1956. (Mimeographed report)

additional two years. During this period full time was to be devoted to the critical problem of the identification of basic science content.

In the process of the original study the basic science facts and understandings were called science principles and concepts. To clarify this terminology the following operational definitions were adopted.

> Science concept: a statement of a generalization based on specific facts.
> Science principle: a statement of a generally accepted fact or a fundamental truth which can be used as a guide to action.

In addition, definitions for nursing concepts and principles were developed.

> Nursing concept: a statement of a generalization based on specific nursing principles.
> Nursing principle: a statement of the application of science principles useful in nursing.

The major purpose of the extended study, then, was the identification of basic science principles and concepts applicable to nursing. The natural sciences were outlined as the physical sciences of chemistry and physics, and the biological sciences of anatomy, physiology (including biochemistry) and microbiology. The social sciences were defined as psychology, sociology and anthropology. No attempt was made to delineate mental hygiene or psychiatric principles. The operational approach was that many psychiatric and most mental hygiene principles are drawn from the basic social sciences, and that the practice of good mental hygiene is the practical application of basic social science principles, in the same way as good physical hygiene is the practical application of natural science principles.

Basic differences between the natural and social sciences and their application to nursing caused a difference in approach to the determination of important principles. The approaches used in the two areas will be described briefly.

HOW THE SCIENCE PRINCIPLES AND THEIR NURSING APPLICATIONS WERE IDENTIFIED

The selection of a method amenable to the identification of science principles important in nursing was somewhat problematic. The sheer bulk of natural science material alone, and the wide variety of nursing practices dependent upon the application of natural science knowledge, presented a formidable barrier to the identification of specific principles. The social sciences, while possessing a bulk of material, do not characteristically lend themselves to statements of principle which can be directly applied. Much of social science knowledge is still in the stage of conceptualization and untested hypotheses. Nursing itself has never been clearly and specifically defined or systematically organized. How then to pursue the task of identifying the nursing application of specific basic science content?

Natural Science

Early in the study it was suggested that the concepts and principles generally taught to nursing students in the various science courses (i.e., anatomy, physiology, physics, chemistry and microbiology) be examined in terms which were applicable to nursing. Although this was a possibility, it seemed that to work in exactly the opposite fashion might prove to be less difficult and more realistic. By the opposite fashion is meant the examination of nursing itself to determine the underlying science facts.

It was this latter approach that led to experimentation with the analysis of common nursing activities such as, for example, measurement of blood pressure and catheterization. These procedures were examined in terms of facts from the natural sciences which, when applied, should result in safe and effective care. Although these analyses proved useful for day-to-day teaching, this method was discontinued for two reasons. In the first place, the specific procedures represented a very limited part of total nursing care. Secondly, the analyses which were completed showed, and not too surprisingly, much repetition of the underlying science principles. For example, the fact that cleanliness inhibits the growth of micro-organisms was found in each analysis; and, whenever an activity involved mucous membrane, one of the applicable principles always set forth was the protective function of a healthy and unbroken membrane.

At this point it was decided that a much broader view of nursing care should be considered in developing a methodology. It was thought that a more comprehensive approach could be made if the nursing care designed to meet the expected physical and medical needs of selected patients were analyzed for underlying science principles.[3] In addition, it was hoped that, if the nursing care were organized carefully and analyzed systematically, there would be relatively little repetition of the principles identified.

The use of this method necessitated the development of individual nursing care plans for hypothetical patients with conditions affecting all the body systems (e.g., the cardiovascular and respiratory systems). When the care plans involving a particular system of the body were completed, the entire section was condensed in such a way as to avoid duplication in the statements of nursing care. The results of the process carried to this point were found to be highly valuable in teaching; however, when some of the completed sections were analyzed, the number of principles identified grew to such an extent that working with them in their interrelated, unorganized state was utterly impractical.

The identification of the important aspects of nursing care proved to be extremely helpful as the study progressed but it was obvious that a method which would provide for the statement of distinctly separate and concise science facts and for as much organization of these facts as possible was of paramount importance. Surely, one way to provide some degree of organization was to direct attention to one area of science at a time.

A review of the analyses accomplished to date revealed that the preponderance of principles came from anatomy and physi-

[3] Physical needs were considered to include such needs as those for the essentials of life (e.g., oxygen) and protection from injury. Medical needs were considered to include such things as special therapies and the observation and reporting of symptoms.

ology. Moreover, it was notable that these principles tended to fall into some broad categories—categories which involved such factors as blood circulation, fluid balance and nutrition. These two observations resulted in the employment of the concept of physiological homeostasis (a favorable internal environment) as a basis for the determination of principles from anatomy and physiology. If the physical nursing care of patients is directed toward either the maintenance or the restoration of homeostasis, this concept should be an excellent organizing factor for the identification of many useful principles.

The first step was to extract elements of homeostasis which could be studied separately. Ten elements were identified as being essential to the maintenance of a constant internal environment of an individual and each of these ten was stated as a sub-concept of homeostasis. The ten sub-concepts dealt with factors such as oxygen, blood pressure and electrolyte balance. In addition to these essential elements there are a number of body functions which, although perhaps not primary components of homeostasis, can be considered to be intimately associated with it. Locomotion and perception of external stimuli are examples of this type of function. The significance of functions such as these led to the formulation of seven more sub-concepts which were added to the original ten.

After the seventeen sub-concepts had been stated, each sub-concept was studied in terms of its embodiment of major facts from anatomy and physiology and, at the same time, its application to nursing. The process required two associated activities. The nursing care related to each sub-concept had to be identified and then analyzed for the underlying science knowledge. Practically simultaneously, anatomy and physiology content related to the sub-concept was reviewed and facts which seemed to be applicable to nursing were selected. One activity supplemented the other.

As the material was developed, no attempt was made to associate specific science principles with each of the nursing activities. Instead, the material was prepared in sections; statements of nursing care related to each sub-concept were made, and these were followed by the principles which were considered to underlie that nursing care. Because the human body is a whole functioning unit, the placement of the facts about structure and function into separate sections proved a difficult and perhaps impossible task. It seemed that the most important thing was to have each fact stated somewhere in the seventeen sections. Repetition was purposely avoided. In many instances cross-references were made in the nursing care sections, and the implication was that the science principles in the one section were applicable also in the other sections.

It probably should be mentioned here that there were variations in the degree of specificity of the statements of the science content. An attempt was made to keep the levels of the statements somewhat similar all the way through, but greater emphasis was placed on trying to state the facts in such a way that they could have meaning to a nurse and be guides to action. All the many details which are sometimes involved in a single broadly-stated fact were not included, and generalizations were not made to the extent that applications of them would become a puzzle. The former was not a purpose of the study and the latter would have resulted in useless material.

Elements of pathology were occasionally included among the statements of anatomy and physiology facts. It was thought that the amount of pathology should be limited, but there were times when certain aspects of disease became important enough to the applications of the principles of physiology that including these aspects seemed worth while.

After each of the sections of nursing care and related principles had been completed, the nursing care was reviewed and criticized by both a medical specialist and a committee of clinical nursing instructors. This committee was called the Natural Science Committee, and its membership was made up of representatives of all clinical areas in nursing. The science principles were reviewed and criticized by a physiologist. Changes in each of the sections were made as recommended by these people.

After the identification of the anatomy and physiology principles had been completed, the nursing care was analyzed for underlying principles from both physics and chemistry. A few of the principles of chemistry, though not directly applicable to nursing care, contributed to the intelligent application of some of the physiology principles. Members of the Natural Science Committee reviewed all the statements formulated; a professor of chemistry criticized the chemistry principles. Changes in the statements were made as recommended, and the principles were added to the previously prepared seventeen sections. Because there were comparatively few of these statements and because it seemed simpler to do so, these principles were repeated in each section from which they were identified.

A nursing principle which appeared in one of the sections of nursing care provided the basis for the identification of important principles from microbiology. The nursing care was concerned with the protection of patients from microbial injury. Again, the nursing care had to be identified along with the underlying science principles and the method used was identical to that which had been employed with the anatomy and physiology sections. Members of the Natural Science Committee and a pathologist reviewed and criticized the nursing care and a medical microbiologist did the same with the science. Changes were made as recommended.

At this stage of the study it became apparent that further identification of important science principles was not possible during the time remaining. Many more principles of science might have been identified through the analyses of nursing responsibilities related to drug administration, diagnostic tests, special therapies and specific nursing procedures utilized to achieve such objectives as providing for comfort, safety and the essentials of life.

After the eighteen sections of nursing care and related science principles had been completed, the total material was given to a jury for evaluation. Six nurse educators in different parts of the country, known to have particular interest in one or more of the natural sciences, were asked to review and criticize the material.

At no time during the development of the material did any person other than the author scrutinize the nursing and the science together for the purpose of ascertaining that the selected principles of science underlie the nursing care. For this reason one major request made of the jury members was that they review each complete section and evaluate the relatedness of the nursing and the science. In addition to this task, they were asked to appraise the nursing care and the science principles in terms of their agreement with the statements. They were asked also to offer suggestions for additional nursing and science principles which they felt should be included and were encouraged to make general comments about the material as a whole. Their responses were used to reorganize, delete and correct the material for final presentation.

Social Sciences

Since social sciences are concerned with human behavior without respect to a specific physiological illness or to treatment or nursing procedures, it did not seem expedient to analyze nursing care plans or nursing procedures to determine social science principles. Such plans and procedures are usually oriented toward physical care or toward the mechanics of carrying out a procedure. Any psycho-social aspects of care which might be appended to such plans or procedures would have had to be stated in broad, relatively meaningless terms, such as "provide reassurance" or "avoid embarrassment."

The possibility of analyzing social science texts, outlines or other reference materials was also ruled out as a possible methodology. It would be difficult to arrive at defensible criteria for the selection and/or ruling out of concepts and principles, as found in current textbooks, which would have particular relevance to nursing. It also would be extremely difficult to develop a framework from which to review the diverse theories and approaches expounded in contemporary sociological literature. One finds a wide variety of theoretical approaches to man's individual and collective behavior, and not all theories are mutually compatible. This lack of agreement was especially crucial to the study when choices had to be made regarding terminology. The problem of terminology will be discussed later with particular reference to some of the concepts and principles included in the social science section of Part II.

After some consideration of available methods, it was decided that an analysis of actual patient-nurse situations might be the most profitable initial approach. Such a method could provide information about the kinds of psycho-social problems which patients actually encounter in the course of illness and hospitalization, irrespective of the presenting complaint, physiological illness or the resulting care and treatment. Material collected in this way also might help to circumvent one of the major complaints about the use of social science concepts in teaching nursing students—the difficulty in arriving at specific principles to guide the nurse's behavior.

With these considerations in mind, an adaptation of Flanagan's[4] "Critical Incident Technique" was chosen as the primary means of collecting source material for the statement of principles. This method provided for the collection of descriptions of patient and nurse behavior in operationally defined critical situations. Critical incidents were defined as nurse-patient situations in which patients were either helped (a positive situation) or harmed (a negative situation) by some action of a nursing team member. The benefit or harm to the patient was described in terms of the patient's observable reaction to the situation.

Descriptions of nurse-patient situations were collected from nurses who were involved in giving patient care or in supervising patient care on medical, surgical and obstetrical[5] services of four large general hospitals. The nurses were asked to describe incidents in which they had recently been involved or which they had recently observed. These incidents then were analyzed in terms of the social science principles which seemed to be inherent in the situation.

There were certain assumptions, beliefs and other criteria which guided the analysis of the situations and the statement of principles. Some of these assumptions or beliefs are as follows:

[4] Flanagan, John C.: The Critical Incident Technique, Psychological Bulletin, Vol. 51, No. 4, July 1954, pp. 327-358.

[5] Since one of the hospitals did not have an obstetrical unit, material in this area was supplemented by a study using similar methods for the same purpose.

Rose, Patricia: The Identification of Psychiatric Principles Inherent in the Nursing Care of a Selected Group of Maternity Patients (unpublished Masters thesis, Univ. Washington, 1958).

Assumption: That the human being cannot survive as a psychologically healthy social being (even though he may physiologically survive) unless certain required conditions prevail. It was further assumed that these conditions include both internal (psychological) and external (socio-cultural) factors which have a reciprocal relationship.

Assumption: That the human organism functions as a total unit, implying that physiological homeostasis is affected by psycho-social factors, and that psycho-social homeostasis is affected by physiological factors.

Assumption: That the person who seeks medical attention, and subsequently receives nursing care, for a disturbance of physiological function will require, and has a right to expect, attention and care in the area of psycho-social function if he is to receive maximum benefit from medical and nursing care.

The collection and analysis of situations represented an attempt to arrive at some of the factors which influence the human being's psycho-social equilibrium while he is in a situation which requires nursing care.

A further belief is stated in terms of nursing responsibility. It was held that a person who is in the situation described by the above assumptions comes within the province of nursing responsibility. Moreover, the nurse must necessarily have the understandings and the abilities which permit her to assist the person toward achievement of psycho-social equilibrium whenever equilibrium is disturbed, or likely to be disturbed, as a result of the situation.

The terms "psycho-social equilibrium" and "psychological homeostasis" were used, even though they seemed to be in disfavor in current sociological literature. It is here that we begin to have trouble with terminology. Equilibrium and homeostasis, as used in the natural sciences, can be defined with far greater scientific accuracy than when applied to social science material. Relatively speaking, other terms would be equally difficult to define, would meet with equal disfavor from some readers, and would be less useful for present purposes.

In the social science material in Part II the term "homeostasis" refers to the tendency of an organism to seek and maintain relatively stable conditions of existence. In the physical sciences, homeostasis has a restricted meaning, implying the *internal* stability of an organism as maintained by self-regulatory mechanisms. For this study, the term was usefully expanded to include psychological and social factors which influence human stability and the individual and collective actions man may take to establish and maintain relative homeostasis.

The common dictionary definition was used for the term "equilibrium." This definition implies a state of balance or even adjustment between opposing forces, influences, interests, etc. of any kind. As used in the social science material, equilibrium and homeostasis are complimentary conditions toward which the human being strives in his attempts to exist in relative safety and comfort. These two terms provided a useful frame of reference for looking at a human being as a total entity and for correlating physiological and psycho-social components of patient care.

In the analysis of situations, several questions were asked. Why was a helpful action taken? Why was it helpful? Why was a particular action harmful? What knowledge or understanding, if possessed by the nursing team member, would most likely have led to the helpful action or prevented the harmful action or lack of action? Answers to these questions were stated in terms of basic science principles.

Here again there was difficulty with terminology. The term "principle" was used to describe the statements derived from the analysis. In common practice this term has been used rather loosely to denote any currently believed "fact" or idea, with or without scientific validation. In the science fields principles have a much more restricted meaning. In the area of the social sciences, strictly scientific principles which have been proven by testing are few and far between! In order to avoid as much controversy as possible, both the terms "principle" and "hypothesis" have been used to designate the statements arrived at in the process of incident analysis. The term "hypothesis" refers to a tentative theory or supposition provisionally adopted to explain certain facts and to guide in the investigation of others, or something assumed or conceded for the purpose of argument or action.

The author was assisted in the process of screening and analyzing incidents by a group of School of Nursing faculty members representative of all clinical areas in nursing. This group is referred to as the Social Science Committee. Throughout the entire period of study, this committee functioned both as an informal jury to guide the decisions of the author and as a work group to analyze situations and formulate statements of principle.

For the incidents analyzed, there were 432 separate statements of principle or hypothesis. Many of these statements reappeared for numerous situations in the same or slightly different form. There was considerable overlapping and duplication in the original statements, and they were at all levels of generality from broad conceptual statements to statements of specific fact. A few of the statements were in terms of nursing principles and concepts rather than science principles and concepts. After the incidents had been analyzed, the statements were categorized and organized as presented in Part II. When the organization had been completed, a Related Nursing Care Section was developed to demonstrate the relationship of the basic social sciences to nursing. The material then was critically reviewed by two members of the University of Washington Department of Psychology.

After corrections had been made, the material was submitted to a group of six additional social scientists for review. This group included one additional psychologist, two sociologists and three anthropologists. With the exception of the anthropologists, all of the reviewers had had some experience in the health science fields. They were asked to consider the principles and hypotheses from the standpoint of: (1) the truth of the statements, (2) the relevance of sub-statements to major statements and (3) the relevance of the nursing section to the science sections. The responses of the reviewers were used to reorganize, delete and correct the material for final use.

CHAPTER II: *Potential Usefulness of the Principles for Nursing Education*

During the process of developing the science principles and nursing care presented in Part II it was inevitable that the authors should spend some of their time dreaming about how the material could be of value to themselves, to other instructors of nursing or, possibly, to science teachers who work with nursing students. One of the most exciting features of identifying the principles has been the imagination shown by persons who participated in the study in considering the various ways in which these principles might be utilized in teaching.

The following suggestions are offered to the reader as possible means of utilizing the material. It is hoped and expected that instructors will discover many other helpful functions. In the discussion which follows, the natural and social sciences have been separated to some extent because of differences in content, and combined to some extent because both underlie comprehensive nursing care.

For the sake of having some kind of organizational pattern for the consideration of possible uses for the statements of nursing and the related science principles, the authors have selected a recognized method of curriculum development to serve this purpose. The method selected advocates the following:

1. Definition of objectives, including content and behavior.
2. Planning of learning experiences to attain these objectives.
3. Selection and organization of learning experiences.
4. Evaluation of attainment of the objectives.

DEFINITION OF OBJECTIVES

It can be assumed that one major objective of any nursing curriculum will have to do with the ability to perform effectively the nursing care of patients. An important question stemming from this general objective is "What is effective nursing care?" An attempt to answer this question leads naturally to a qualitative analysis of nursing care—an analysis which takes into consideration the major aspects of nursing as well as the means for accomplishing nursing care to the desired end of patient well-being.

Because the life of an individual is dependent upon the maintenance of a constant internal environment (physiological homeostasis) and because in disease that internal environment is threatened and/or changed, the maintenance and restoration of homeostasis are primary nursing goals. Similarly, the well-being and adequate adjustment of man to life situations are dependent upon the maintenance of psychological homeostasis. Because illness and hospitalization, whether due primarily to a disturbance of physiological function or not, disturb the total pattern of the individual's satisfaction of psycho-social needs, the nurse must be concerned with the maintenance and restoration of psychological homeostasis. The analysis of the nursing care of patients in terms of the requirements of physiological homeostasis is essentially what can be found in Chapter III of Part II. Chapter IV of Part II contains statements of nursing action related to the identified social science principles which have direct bearing on the achievement and maintenance of psychological homeostasis. If the statements of nursing care in these two chapters actually do present major aspects of physical and psychological nursing care, one should be able to use them in the process of defining objectives—objectives related to: (1) providing for physical and psychological comfort, (2) providing for the essentials of life such as oxygen, fluid balance and emotional security, (3) providing for protection from mechanical, chemical, physical, microbial or psychological injury and (4) providing for the observation of deviations from normal physiological and psychological function and the appropriate communication of these deviations to other members of the health team.

It has been pointed out that completely stated objectives contain two essential components: some indication of the behavior which is desired and some indication of an area of content to which that behavior is related. Objectives concerned with the physical and psychological nursing care of patients can be stated readily in this manner. Following are two examples of the development of objectives from the natural and social science material. In the examples, a broad objective was identified and analyzed to ascertain specific objectives inherent in the broad statement.

Natural Science: Over-all Objective

To perform nursing care which serves to maintain the body temperature within a normal range.

Primary Analysis

1. To be able to observe the signs and symptoms of:
   A. A normal body temperature.
   B. An elevated body temperature.
   C. A lowered body temperature.

2. To be able to perform activities designed to:
   A. Measure the body temperature.
   B. Lower the elevated body temperature.
   C. Elevate a lowered body temperature.
   D. Meet physiological needs associated with abnormal body temperatures.

3. To be able to communicate with others relative to:
   A. The signs and symptoms of a normal, elevated or lowered body temperature.
   B. The performance of procedures for measuring body temperature, lowering or elevating body temperature, and meeting physiological needs associated with abnormal body temperatures.

Continued Analysis

1. To understand normal regulation of body temperature.
2. To understand possible causes of deviations in temperature regulation and their nursing implications.
3. To understand physiological changes which accompany an elevated or a lowered body temperature.
4. To be able to use the special senses for the purpose of determining the temperature of an individual and any accompanying physiological changes.
5. To be able to apply principles of science in:
   A. Using equipment for measuring body temperature.
   B. Performing various procedural methods designed to maintain or restore normal body temperature, such as:
      (1) Adjustment of external environmental temperature.
      (2) Adjustment of coverings and physical activity.
      (3) Application of heat.
      (4) Removal of heat.
      (5) Administration of drugs.
   C. Performing various functions relative to changes in physiology which occur, or may occur, when there is abnormal body temperature. Such functions might be concerned with:
      (1) Fluid balance.
      (2) Nutrition.
      (3) Care of skin and mucous membranes.
6. To be able to report and record appropriately information relative to body temperature.
7. To be able to teach others relative to:
   A. Basic understandings about body temperature.
   B. Measurement of body temperature.
   C. Important observations relative to deviations from normal body temperature.
   D. Simple technics of regulating body temperature.

E. Simple functions relative to fluid intake, dietary variations and care of the skin and mucous membranes when there are marked temperature changes.

It will be noted that the over-all objective involves one of the sub-concepts of homeostasis; namely, that "there is a definite temperature range for efficient cellular functioning and proper enzymatic activity." The nursing care and underlying science principles related to this sub-concept can be found in Section H of Chapter III.

Social Science: Over-all Objective

To take action which will assist the patient to acquire or maintain the approval of others, or to prevent disapproval from others, in his socio-cultural environment.

Primary Analysis

1. To make observations regarding:
   A. Patient behavior which indicates that he receives adequate approval from others.
   B. Patient behavior which indicates a disturbance of psychological equilibrium due to lack of approval or to disapproval.
   C. Patient behavior which demonstrates the patient's attempts to acquire approval in satisfactory or unsatisfactory ways.
   D. Patient behavior which might cause disapproval or lack of approval.
   E. Factors in the patient's life situation which influence the receiving or withholding of approval or the demonstration of approval.

2. To analyze and interpret the observed data to determine:
   A. The relative satisfaction or dissatisfaction of the patient's need for approval in his current life situation.
   B. The sources of disturbance or interference with the satisfaction of the patient's need for approval.
   C. The necessity and/or feasibility of nursing action to

help the patient satisfy his need for approval in his current life situation.

D. The extent of nursing responsibility in assisting the patient toward satisfaction of his need for approval.

E. The necessity and/or feasibility of referring the patient to other sources of assistance.

3. To take specific nursing action aimed at:
   A. Removing, eliminating or changing factors in the current situation which cause the patient to feel disapproval or lack of approval.
   B. Providing an environment and/or experiences which will contribute to the patient's feeling of being approved.
   C. Providing the patient with psychological support as he works through adjustive problems relative to receiving approval or avoiding disapproval.
   D. Helping the patient to change behavior which interferes with receiving approval or causes disapproval.

4. To communicate with other members of the health team regarding:
   A. Patient behavior which indicates a disturbance of psychological equilibrium due to lack of approval or to disapproval from others and the causes of the disturbance.
   B. A plan of care which will assist the patient in the satisfaction of his need of approval.

Continued Analysis

1. An understanding of and ability to recognize human behavior which indicates a state of psychological disequilibrium due to lack of approval or to disapproval from others in one's socio-cultural environment.

2. An understanding of the dynamics of human behavior relative to the satisfaction of this particular need.

3. An understanding of the relationship between psychological equilibrium and physiological homeostasis, as demonstrated by lack of satisfaction of this need.

4. An understanding of the socio-cultural influences on the satisfaction of this need in general and in the current specific situation.

5. An understanding of personality growth and development patterns which influence the satisfaction of this need.

6. An understanding of and ability to function within the nursing role in the satisfaction of this need.

7. A knowledge of additional sources of assistance in satisfying the patient's need and how to utilize these sources when necessary.

8. An understanding of and ability to apply socio-psychological principles in establishing an environment which will:
   A. Eliminate or reduce sources of disapproval.
   B. Provide for or encourage opportunities for the patient to receive approval from others.
   C. Provide the patient with psychological support and encouragement when he is working through potentially traumatic problems relative to approval or disapproval.
   D. Assist the patient to learn new behaviors or modify behaviors which will contribute to a feeling of approval or the elimination of disapproval.

It will be noted that the over-all objective involves one of the sub-concepts relative to psychological homeostasis—"the approval of others in one's socio-cultural environment is necessary for psychological homeostasis". The nursing care and underlying principles related to this sub-concept can be found in Chapter IV, Section C.

In each of the primary analyses of the above examples, major skills (observational, technical and communicative) involved in the nursing care were identified along with a general description of the nursing content. The more specific objectives stated in the continued analyses not only include reference to these major skills but also contain some degree of information about the knowledge which underlies the effective performance of these skills and a more complete description of nursing activities involved in the skills with respect to their importance in attaining the over-all objective.

The skills, the knowledge and the specific nursing activities included in the foregoing examples are either stated or implied in the material contained in Chapters III and IV of Part II. It can be seen that this material does not provide complete and final answers to the questions of *what* skills and *what* knowledge should be taught to nursing students. It does, however, provide a basis for determining some of the behaviors and some of the content toward which clinical nursing instructors should be guiding their students. Other objectives similar to those presented here can be identified from the analysis of the natural and social science material.

IDENTIFICATION, SELECTION AND ORGANIZATION OF LEARNING EXPERIENCES

The determination of possible learning experiences which could be developed to attain desired objectives stems quite naturally from a careful examination of the objectives. If understanding is involved, the nursing student must have access through such media as lectures, laboratory sessions, informal discussions, textbooks and guided observations of the facts which are essential to the understanding. The same is true if the objective concerns the application of science principles. The student should be given an opportunity to learn the science principles before or during the teaching of the nursing care which involves the application of those principles.

The science principles identified in this study as being important for a nurse to understand and be able to apply can be used as a partial answer to the question of what science should be taught. Identification of additional facts can be accomplished through the analysis of specific observational and technical skills involved in physical nursing care through the analysis of specific diagnostic tests and therapeutic procedures in which the nurse participates or which she should be able to interpret. Additional facts also can be identified through the analysis of specific patient problems in the area of social and psychological adjustment when such problems are encountered in the nurse-patient situation.

The ability to observe signs and symptoms, the ability to apply principles of science in the performance of nursing care, and the ability to perform tasks with some degree of manual dexterity can be developed only through practice. This implies that one responsibility of the clinical instructor is the planning of student experiences so that problems involving these skills are provided. Discussion of teaching methods for the development of understandings and skills is not within the scope of this book. However, some general considerations of the selection and organization of learning experiences utilizing the identified science principles and associated nursing care will be included.

One type of decision which every clinical instructor in nursing faces concerns the choice of patients for students to care for during clinical practice. There are many factors to be taken into consideration in this selection process, as for example: the individual learning needs of each student, the theoretical preparation which the student has, and the need for new learning pertaining to a particular type of nursing problem. Now that the trend in nursing education seems to be toward decreasing the time that students spend in the bedside practice of patient care, this selection process has become increasingly significant. The use of more effective teaching methods with emphasis upon specific, selected learning goals has shown that it is possible to shorten the length of time a student devotes to clinical experiences. The objectives for such learning experiences must be clearly defined, and the experiences themselves must be carefully planned. Following are some examples of how the principles contained in Chapters III and IV can be used in the identification, selection and organization of learning experiences.

Natural Sciences

The statements of nursing care included in Chapter III can be helpful in selecting patients for the purpose of teaching physical nursing care. If the teaching of nursing proceeds through a consideration of the major physiological problems which people have, the lists of medical, surgical, obstetrical and psychiatric conditions included in the first nursing care statement in each section can provide a source of guidance in the selection of patients who have, or are likely to have, those particular physiological problems. For instance, upon the examination of the conditions related to the body's requirement for adequate oxygen it will be noted that patients with many different conditions might provide good learning experiences. The instructor might select a patient who is unconscious or one with a severe head injury, a lung tumor, pneumonia, asthma, ascites, or a patent ductus arteriosus. Which patient the instructor selects would or should be decided not only on the basis of the type of respiratory problem involved but also on the basis of other problems which the patient presents and how well prepared the student is in the nursing care of patients with these other problems.

The care of a patient with an acute, uncomplicated attack of bronchial asthma probably would involve the administration of certain types of drugs and, possibly, oxygen. The care of a patient with pneumonia might involve the administration of antibiotic drugs, the administration of oxygen, special positioning, isolation technics and the management of fever. The care of a patient with ascites might involve special positioning, the administration of certain drugs, various nutritional problems, problems of fluid and electrolyte balance and assisting a doctor with a paracentesis.

These last observations lead to a further consideration of the teaching of nursing care in such a way as to proceed from the simple to the complex. A careful review of the nursing care included in Chapter III offers an opportunity to determine various levels of nursing care. That is, through the analysis of the nursing care in each section, along with the related science principles, one can identify comparatively basic, uncomplicated nursing care, moderately complicated nursing care, and complex nursing care. One can identify the types of problems patients have which require these differing levels of care.

Would it be good judgment to have a beginning student care for a patient with a head injury? Such a patient might have problems which involve circulation, respiration, nutrition, fluid balance, pH, temperature regulation, elimination, motor and sensory activity, the skin, infection and behavior. In the same vein, how fruitful would it be to have a student near graduation, for the purpose of learning physical nursing care, care for a patient who was having an uneventful convalescence following an appendectomy?

Bruno[6] has experimented with a method for determining levels of complexity in nursing care as this complexity is revealed by the analysis of nursing care into specific activities and the numbers of related science principles. In her study she chose two functional areas of nursing care: the positioning of patients and provision for their physical activities. The nursing care was identified through the analysis of five nursing textbooks and combined into large categories concerned with good body alignment and the positions and physical activities commonly used when there are various physiological problems. The nursing care then was examined in an effort to identify principles of anatomy, physiology and physics which were closely related to the many nursing activities. The science principles stated in some parts of the material in Chapter III were used for this purpose.

In the analysis of the data, Bruno divided the nursing care and principles into different categories determined by the extent to which a patient was able to meet his own needs for positioning and physical activity. She then totalled the science principles associated with the major nursing activities. The degree of complexity of nursing care was consdered to be indicated by (1) the numbers of nursing activities involved in achieving certain goals relative to positioning and physical activities and (2) the numbers of science principles which were related to each nursing activity. Similar studies could be done in other functional areas of nursing, using the statements of nursing care and underlying science principles in Chapter III.

[6] Bruno, Pauline: A Determination and Examination of Nursing Measures and Related Science Principles Which Pertain to Positioning of Patients and Providing for their Physical Activities. (Unpublished post-Masters research investigation supported by a Research Fellowship [NF-7641] from the Division of Nursing Resources of the Public Health Service.) Univ. Washington, 1958.

Social Sciences

The social sciences as applied to general nursing practice are for several reasons less amenable to the consistent selection and organization of learning experiences than the natural sciences. With the exception of neuro-psychiatric or psychiatric illness, the patient's primary presenting problem is physiological in nature so that at all times, in health agencies used for teaching, one can find problems relative to the eighteen sections outlined in Chapter III. Since the patient asks for help with his physiological problems, the diagnosis or identification of the problem area is made by the physician, and the instructor will locate patients who will provide suitable experience for learning physical care at all levels of complexity. While every patient will have some psycho-social disturbance by virtue of being a totally reacting organism, the nature and the severity of the disturbance will vary with each individual patient regardless of his presenting problem. This does not encourage the use of a predetermined organizational pattern for the selection of learning experiences according to major psycho-social needs. Furthermore, an identification of the patient's problems in this area, being secondary to his presenting complaint, is not a part of the formal diagnosis; and such an identification occurs, if at all, during the ensuing process of physical nursing care. Unless the problem is outstanding, the identification of such problems usually is left to the discretion of the nurse and seldom receives medical attention or orders for care.

In some ways the selection of learning experiences in the social science areas is helped rather than hindered by these factors. If we can assume that all patients will have some degree of disturbance of psycho-social equilibrium as a result of physical illness and hospitalization, then we also can assume that every patient will provide the student with an opportunity to learn and to apply social science principles. If this is so, the instructor's problem is not so much one of selection and organization, but of identification and effective utilization of constant opportunity and careful guidance of the student in successive learning experiences. The successive experiences provide natural opportunity for increasing the depth of understanding and increasing skill in meeting problem situations which have to do with the patient's psycho-social adjustment.

It is the opinion of the authors that it would be impossible to avoid *potential* learning experiences, at all levels of complexity, involving social science principles regardless of the rationale for the selection and organization of learning experiences where patients are involved. It is in the failure of the instructor to recognize and utilize experiences that we encounter the lack of economical use of student learning time and capabilities. For example, let us consider the patient's need for satisfying relationships with others. Whatever the patient's reason for seeking medical care, his need for satisfying relationships is not left at home. He will, if he is hospitalized, experience some feeling of separation, of being alone. Unless health team members make attempts to prevent it, or unless it can be achieved through good physical care, he will feel uncared for. Because he is in an environment which includes many other people, usually strangers, he will have an increased need for the acceptance and approval of these people, upon whom he must depend for his continued health and well-being. Since every patient has had different growth and development experiences, each will demonstrate individual differences in the way he attempts to meet these needs; and since every patient is a member of some socio-cultural group, his behavior will indicate the influence of his particular group in meeting these needs. Further, the patient is in a new social situation where he will have to learn the roles and functions of those around him and how he fits into the social structure of hospital life.

Unless the instructor deliberately avoided patients who demonstrated intensified, chronic or exaggerated needs in these areas, the law of averages would make it impossible for the student not to encounter patients who demonstrate a range from highly satisfactory to acutely unsatisfactory relationships with others. The only problem in the deliberate selection of experiences for learning increasingly complex psychological nursing care is encountered when there are extreme degrees of psycho-social need. If the student is only beginning to learn the principles involved in, for example, helping the patient to achieve and maintain satisfying relationships with others, it is easy enough to avoid assignment to patients whose disturbances in this area are so great as to cause behavior which deviates widely from normal. Such experiences can be planned for later in the program, when the student may be assigned to a psychiatric unit, in which the patient's presenting problem is in this area. Similar examples could be given for all of the identified social science material in Chapter IV. The crucial factor in guiding the student's learning of skill in applying social science principles is in the instructor's recognition of constant opportunity and in her deliberate plans to capitalize on natural resources. It seems quite reasonable to say that learning under such circumstances would be most effective because it would help the student to recognize the interdependence of all aspects of human functions, regardless of the specific acute problems.

If the instructor feels that it is necessary to have an organized outline or plan, she could utilize the identified principles to formulate a check list for herself, together with a more formalized plan for teaching according to the kinds of problems that students are most likely to encounter at various stages in their growth and development as nursing students. For example, the young student encounters her first problem in human relations when she meets a patient face to face and must communicate with him both for purposes of observation and comfort for herself and the patient. Emphasis on learning in this first experience, together with formal classes or ward conferences, might well be directed toward acquiring a beginning skill in communication. As the student is able to be comfortable in simple verbal communication with a patient, further guidance and conference time could be planned to increase her understanding of the total communication process and to use communication for therapeutic purposes. This implies the need for additional understanding of the dynamics of verbal and non-verbal communication, the use of symbols in communication, the dynamics of perception and some understanding of specific problems which can be solved through effective communication.

In addition, by reviewing the plan for the teaching of physical care, the instructor can foresee other problems which are likely to occur with regularity. For example, while students are having clinical experiences related to the maintenance of an adequate supply of oxygen, it is almost certain that they will encounter acute fear on the part of the patient because of the threat to his life. At this time, the instructor can plan to help the students learn some of the dynamics of behavior related to fear and some of the skills, based on principles, that the nurse needs in order to minimize fear. This method of organization has the advantage of being based on student motivation to solve the problems with which she is immediately faced.

The foregoing has covered a few ideas pertaining primarily to the identification, selection and organization of learning experiences in clinical nursing practice. Perhaps a few additional suggestions can be made regarding the selection and organization of learning experiences which are largely theoretical in nature.

The discussion which follows has been limited to suggestions for helping nursing students to learn or to apply science principles. It is the sincere belief of the authors that a professional nurse should base her nursing care on science principles. The ability to apply such principles in giving nursing care enables the nurse to interpret and to follow medical orders intelligently, to perform and to adapt nursing activities effectively, and to be creative in the planning and the execution of the nursing care of the individual patient. This ability helps to prevent rigidity in thinking and acting; it frees her from continual dependence upon others for solving her nursing problems; it frees her from the monotony of repetitious nursing activities which she might perform according to routine rather than reason. In short, this ability provides the nurse with one means of becoming a truly professional person.

The usual pattern of teaching science to nursing students is the teaching of it before the student has her clinical practice; that is, before she has direct contact with patients. A supposed advantage of this pattern is that the student comes to the clinical nursing instructor possessing the important facts of anatomy, physiology, physics, chemistry, microbiology, sociology and psychology which she can then proceed to apply in learning and performing nursing actions. This seems to be an ideal method but in actual practice this pattern sometimes does not work. There are many possible reasons for this. The instructors in the various science fields may not be familiar with what aspects of the science are important in nursing; or they may be familiar with it but must teach a science course which cannot be directed toward the specific learning needs of nursing students. The clinical instructors may be weak in their own science preparation, causing difficulty in the integration of science into the teaching of nursing. The nursing instructor may not believe that the ability to apply science principles in solving nursing problems is an objective of nursing education, or she may not know what science content to integrate or what methods to use for successful integration. She also may be unaware of how much science content, or what specific science content, the student has had prior to her clinical experience. The students themselves may have learned relatively little science while taking the pre-clinical courses in an academic setting. They may have forgotten much of the memorized science content before they reach the clinical experience, or they may need to learn additional science content. Not infrequently they will need considerable guidance and practice in solving problems through systematic thinking which requires the application of principles of science.

Let us look at a few of the possible ways in which the natural and social science material could be helpful in overcoming some of the difficulties mentioned in the foregoing paragraph. If the instructors of science courses are available for conferences with the clinical nursing instructor and are amenable to such conferences, the clinical instructor can seek information about the science course content as presently being taught. She could inform the science instructor of the nursing students' needs for specific science content. She also might work with the science teacher in determining discrepancies between the science content taught and the science content needed in nursing and decide who will teach what science content in the future.

The material in Chapters III and IV could be used by clinical instructors to identify weak spots in their own knowledge of science which they need to strengthen if they are to do integrative teaching. The material also might serve as a guide in thinking about how science can be applicable to nursing. It also seems possible that instructors could use the material in planning learning experiences for students which would help them in recalling important science content, learning additional science content and applying science principles to nursing. Following are some examples of how the principles can be used in helping students to recall or learn science content and to apply principles of science to the solution of nursing problems.

Review or Learning of Natural Science Content

Study guides can be prepared for students for use in the review of science content. These study guides can direct the student rather pointedly to specific knowledge which she should have readily available. There is a decided difference between suggesting that students review the anatomy and physiology of the cardiovascular system and suggesting that they review such well-defined content as factors which affect blood pressure, how the circulation of blood is accomplished in the human body and how the clotting of blood occurs. A student could study for a week with the first assignment and not be well prepared for her clinical nursing experience. In the second assignment, she could focus her studying on science knowledge pertinent to her nursing care.

Class time can be planned for the express purpose of helping students to broaden and deepen their knowledge of science content in preparation for nursing classes. For instance, it is generally recognized that students tend to have a difficult time understanding the anatomy and physiology of the nervous system. While studying such a complex subject, it is not uncommon for a student to become so engrossed with details during her introduction to the content that the more general understandings which will be useful to her in nursing are lost by the wayside. Therefore, it may be desirable to devote class time to the discussion of important aspects of neuro-anatomy and neuro-physiology.

Formal classes and/or informal discussions which are planned to explore specific nursing problems also provide a means of helping students to recall science content. In this case, the application of knowledge is considered in addition to a review of the knowledge needed.

Study guides can be made specific enough to direct the student's study toward important new science content. Classes can be planned exclusively for the purpose of introducing new content. It may be desirable to ask resource people such as science instructors to teach this sort of class. Because many courses in general microbiology required as part of nursing curricula may not include some of the microbiology principles which are most useful to a nurse, this type of class may be indicated to teach microbiology content relevant to nursing.

If the amount of new content to be taught is not extensive, it can be nicely integrated along with the usual classes and informal discussions. If the classes and the discussions are planned and conducted in such a way that the basic "whys" are an integral part of any discussion, new science content fits quite naturally into place. If going back to basic science for these reasons is not a common practice in teaching, such integration will require special attention.

Review or Learning of Social Science Content

One of the most effective ways for reviewing or learning social science content is through the use of references and questions pertaining to specific patient problems as the student encounters such problems in clinical practice. Theoretically, the most effective learning could be achieved if the individual student could be guided toward reference reading which would be in accord with the specific patient problem which she is concerned with at any given time. Practically, there is seldom a high enough ratio of instructors to students to make this entirely possible. The authors have found that group discussion of prepared problems, accompanied by reading assignments, has been useful for purposes of both review and new learning. These prepared problems, or cases, can be constructed on the basis of actual problems which one or more of the students in the group are having to deal with at the time. For example, we can refer to the area of communication as it was discussed in relation to the selection and organization of learning experiences. If one or several of the students are experiencing some difficulty in communicating effectively with their patients, a case could be constructed which would include the common and the specific elements of the actual experiential problem. References could be given for the students to review or read preparatory to the group discussion. If this method is used, there should be some designated time, such as weekly or bi-weekly, for continuity in planning so that each case can build upon previous cases. The social science material as identified in Chapter IV could serve as resource material for planning and construction of case materials and for the selection of references.

Occasionally resource people, lectures or movies will be helpful in acquainting the student with new facts and principles, or in helping the student to look at previous learning in a new light. For example, an anthropologist might be called upon to discuss some of the problems of acculturation, especially as it pertains to health practices.

In addition to group discussion of actual patient problems, the student may be asked to select a nurse-patient situation in which she is involved, to give a written description of the situation with particular emphasis on certain aspects of the situation, and to analyze the situation in terms of social science principles with a justification of her analysis through reference materials. Some of the aspects she might be asked to emphasize are the forms of communication which took place, her own subjective feelings about the patient, behavior of the patient which indicated psychological disequilibrium, or the influence of the various team members on the patient's behavior.

Perhaps one of the most useful methods for helping students to learn social science principles important to nursing is the same method by which the principles and hypotheses in Chapter IV were acquired. If students are helped to identify psychosocial problems of specific patients, and to analyze these problems in terms of underlying science principles, they would need to do less memorization of reference material which might or might not be useful at some later date.

Whatever methods may be used for introduction of new material or the review of previously encountered science content, the important element is the pointing out, or assisting of the student to discover, the relationship of the content to problems of nursing practice. Again, the material in Chapter IV could be useful as a guide for helping students to look for such relationships.

Application of Science Principles

During the original study the authors found that the most effective method for teaching the application of science principles was through the use of problem-solving technics. As might be expected, the more practice the students had in using science to solve nursing problems, the more adept they became in the process. In the use of this teaching method it is important that clinical instructors create an atmosphere, both in the classroom and in the clinical situation, which is conducive to the solution of problems by students. Encouraging students to look at situations analytically is essential. When the instructor continually steps in with a direct and positive answer to a problem, quite naturally the student's ability to solve problems is not allowed to develop.

The natural science and social science material can be helpful in planning learning experiences. Problems which involve science principles can be identified through the examination of the nursing care. Identification of related principles of science can be facilitated by examination of the science material. For example, suppose a clinical instructor wished to plan a class in which the nursing care of an unconscious patient was to be discussed. We know that an unconscious patient requires extensive nursing care because of the patient's dependence upon others for meeting his needs, both physical and psycho-social. One can readily identify the major needs of such a patient and the nursing measures designed to meet these needs through the scanning of the nursing material in all eighteen sections of Chapter III and the related nursing material in the five sections of Chapter IV.

Are there problems related to blood pressure or volume? This may depend upon the cause of the comatose state. It may be that the patient has hypertension or hypotension. What nursing measures are indicated when there is an abnormally high or low blood pressure? If the patient is unable to move himself, the nurse will have to consider maintaining adequate circulation to certain of the body tissues such as muscles and skin. The instructor then may refer to the nursing care related to muscles in Section K and that related to skin in Section L of the natural science material. Are there problems of communication? Does the level of consciousness permit sufficient awareness of surroundings to allow the patient to feel anxious regarding physical care? How do family relationships enter into the nursing care situation? After consideration of these problems, the students could proceed to identify the specific nursing care involved and how this nursing care can be performed effectively.

Following are some of the natural science principles related to the above nursing considerations. They have been extracted from the material in Chapter III, Sections A, K and L.

1. The amount of blood circulating to body parts may be limited by external pressure exerted against blood vessels.
2. Either a marked increase or decrease in the blood supply to the brain can cause loss of consciousness.
3. Postural changes affect arterial blood pressure.
4. Increased muscular activity results in an increase in the blood supply to the active muscles.
5. Fluids flow from an area of higher pressure to one of lower pressure.
6. Major muscles of the body include the flexors and extensors of the toes and fingers; the flexors, extensors and rotators of the feet and hands; the extensors of the legs and thighs; the flexors and extensors of the lower arm, the flexors, extensors and rotators of the upper arm; the supinators and pronators of the forearm; the extensors of the vertebral column; the interscapular muscles and the abdominal musculature.
7. The epidermis of the skin is avascular, nourished by tissue fluid circulation only.
8. Individual skins vary in their resistance to injury.

In the same manner, some of the social science principles can be identified, depending upon the level of consciousness of the patient and his ability to respond. Examples from Chapter IV, Sections A, B and C are:

1. A feeling of comfort and safety in life situations may be achieved by the establishment of familiar routines, behavior patterns, responses from others, etc., which have been experienced as safe and comfortable.
2. Disturbances of equilibrium which result in exaggerated emotional reaction and/or mental dysfunction will decrease the individual's ability to cope with a situation successfully.
3. A feeling of comfort and safety frequently may be achieved through dependence upon others.
4. Clarity, simplicity and lack of threat in the way others approach a confused person, or one who is easily confused, facilitates cooperation between the confused person and others in the environment and the feeling of comfort and safety of the confused person.
5. Actions of others motivated by the anticipation of and attempts to satisfy an individual's needs tends to increase one's feeling of safety and comfort.
6. Non-verbal behavior is used frequently as a means of communication.
7. An individual whose conscious awareness is impaired will need protection from environmental stimulation which may be frightening.

EVALUATION OF THE ATTAINMENT OF OBJECTIVES

If objectives are well defined, the development of evaluation tools to measure the attainment of these objectives is markedly facilitated. The type of evaluative method selected will, of course, depend largely upon the kind of behavior which is to be measured. The discussion of general methods of evaluation is not within the scope of this book; however, suggestions will be made relative to the use of the statements of nursing care and science principles in developing evaluation tools.

There are a number of criteria to take into consideration

when evaluating the nursing care given to patients. Possible criteria include completeness of care, therapeutic effectiveness of care, safety of care for the patient and staff, and physiological and psychological comfort to the patient. All the sections of nursing care included in Chapters III and IV can be used to decide what to look for in relation to such criteria while the instructor evaluates a nursing student's performance.

For paper and pencil tests, test items can be constructed which will measure various aspects of the understanding of and the ability to apply principles of science. The material containing nursing care and related science principles can be of use as a resource for the development of test items concerned with these behaviors.

Essay-type questions can ask that the student compare and contrast the nursing care of two or three patients with fairly similar physiological or psycho-social problems and that she support her answers with known facts. The student also might be asked to describe the nursing care of any patient with a specific physiological or psycho-social problem and to justify this care in terms of science principles. A third type of essay question might ask the student to state the applications of a particular science principle or principles. Another way of using essay questions for this material would be to ask the student to make a choice of nursing actions for a certain situation and then to give reasons for her choice.

Objective-type questions can be constructed to determine both the student's understanding and her ability to apply principles. One type of test experimented with at the University of Washington was called the Application of Sciences Test. Two sets of tests, each with a corresponding part for the natural and social sciences, composed of multiple choice items were constructed. In one set of tests, the student was asked to select proper courses of action for given situations. In the second set, the student was asked to select science principles which would be the best guides to action in given situations. The items were constructed in such a way that the best answer in an item in the first test was based on the principle which would be the best guide for action in an item in the second test. Insofar as was possible, the situations in the associated items were sufficiently different to avoid the possibility of choosing the correct answer on the basis of similarity of items. The second set of tests were given at some time after the first set. Theoretically, such tests can be used to measure not only a student's knowledge but also her ability to apply that knowledge. If she selects the best answers in both associated test items, it may be assumed that she is able to apply the particular science principle involved.

Tschudin,[7] as part of her investigations of students' ability to apply science principles (through the use of the Application of Natural Science Tests) asked that some students, after answering the first test, go back over the test items and state as well as they could the reasons for selecting the answers they chose. The reasons the students gave them were analyzed in terms of whether science principles were utilized, correctly or incorrectly, or whether the answer selected was little more than a guess or based on a rule of thumb.

Construction of any of these kinds of test items can be greatly facilitated by the use of the material in Chapters III and IV. The material can help in identifying important areas within which questions can be developed as well as important points to be included. It also provides a good source of ideas for alternative responses in the case of multiple-choice test items.

. . . .

This chapter was written, not to instruct clinical nursing teachers in the use of the material resulting from the study, but to offer some suggestions for finding ways in which it might be helpful. Suggestions have been made relative to the use of the material for defining objectives, planning, selecting and organizing learning experiences, and evaluating the attainment of objectives. It is the hope of the authors that these suggestions will prove to be helpful in the teaching of nursing students and that instructors will find other practical uses for the material.

[7] Tschudin, Mary S.: A Study of the Relationship Between Nursing Students' Knowledge of Scientific Principles and Their Ability to Apply These Principles in Nursing Situations (Unpublished doctoral thesis, Univ. Washington, 1958).

Part Two

CHAPTER III: *Nursing Care and Underlying Natural Science Principles*

THIS CHAPTER has been divided into two parts. The first contains statements of nursing care and underlying principles from the sciences of anatomy, physiology, physics and chemistry. The nursing care has been limited to that which is directly concerned with seventeen elements of or functions related to physiological homeostasis. The second part contains statements of nursing care which pertain to protection from microbial injury and underlying principles from the science of microbiology. The outline form was used throughout because it provided for the clearest presentation of the extensive material.

All of the sections in the first part were prepared in a like fashion. The nursing care and the science principles in each section are preceded by the statement of the sub-concept of homeostasis to which they are related. The statements of nursing care in each section also have been arranged as similarly as the content allowed. The first two statements always concern the observation and reporting of signs and symptoms. The two statements were separated because of limitations set by the use of outline form. Following these, there are usually statements pertaining to the maintenance of normal structure and function and/or general nursing measures relative to the problem at hand. These are followed by statements related to specific nursing measures which may or should be employed when there is abnormal functioning.

A few comments probably should be inserted here about the observable signs and symptoms which have been listed as reportable. Many physicians might not expect even an experienced professional nurse to be so highly skilled as to recognize all those included. This would be particularly true if the signs and symptoms were subtle. It is doubted that anyone would *object* to a nurse possessing exceptional skill in the area of observation, but teachers of nursing must decide upon the extent to which they emphasize this ability. Needless to say, no matter what observations the nurse is able to make, these are made for the purposes of assisting the doctor and as a basis for the planning of specific nursing care. In most instances the nurse is not called upon to evaluate her observations for the purpose of diagnosing disease conditions. If and when such a function is required, surely she should have had advanced study in this area.

In most instances the principles from anatomy and physiology in the various sections were grouped according to the content and there are sub-headings which designate the content of these groupings.

The principles which are concerned with the protection of patients from microbial injury require little in the way of explanation. It will be noted that the statements of nursing care have been kept fairly general, while the science principles are both general and specific. Specific facts about many of the micro-organisms were included because it was believed that nurses should possess fundamental knowledge about microbial agents which commonly cause disease in man. Many nursing measures will be dependent upon this knowledge. It is quite possible that the reader may disagree with the decision as to which micro-organisms should be included.

Section A: Nursing Care and Science Principles Related to the Volume and Pressure of Circulating Blood.

A. The blood serves as a means of transport for substances to and from the cells, and the volume and pressure of circulating blood must be maintained within certain limits to provide for changing demands of the organs.

NURSING CARE

1. Patients should be observed for signs and symptoms of circulatory problems, and these should be reported. This is of particular importance when the patient has:
   A. A disease condition affecting the heart and/or the blood vessels.
   B. Bleeding or if there is a possibility of bleeding (e.g. post-surgery, following injury to an area of the body which has a relatively large blood supply, abnormal blood clotting, when duodenal or peptic ulcer are suspected or when cancer is suspected).
   C. Been receiving medications which affect the vasomotor mechanisms, heart action or clotting mechanisms.
   D. A relatively large amount of blood in the periphery (e.g. after a hot bath or after exposure to sun).
   E. A rapid loss of plasma (e.g. in burns, generalized allergic response).
   F. Injury or a possibility of injury to the medulla.
   G. A pregnancy or has just delivered.
   H. Severe physical trauma or emotional stress.

I. A cast, dressings, bandages or traction applied.

2. Reportable signs and symptoms of circulatory problems may include:
   A. Observable bleeding from any orifice (nose, mouth, auditory canal, rectum, vagina or urinary meatus), mucous membrane or skin.
      (1) Abnormal vaginal bleeding includes:
         (a) Profuse menstrual bleeding.
         (b) Bleeding between menstrual periods.
         (c) Bleeding other than bloody show during labor.
         (d) Excessive bleeding in the post-partum period.
      (2) Possible signs of abnormal bleeding include:
         (a) Petechiae, ecchymosis.
         (b) Coffee-ground type vomitus.
         (c) Melena.
         (d) Smoky or red-colored urine. (When color changes in urine and/or feces occur, medications which the patient is receiving should be taken into consideration.)
         (e) Failure of the uterus to involute properly after delivery.
      (3) Whenever possible, estimation of the amount of bleeding should be made and total or partial specimens saved for examination.
      (4) Observations for bleeding should be made in any drainage of body fluids and in or around the edges of casts or dressings.
   B. Abnormally high or low blood pressure.
   C. Abnormal pulse rhythm, rate or character. (When there is blood loss or a fall in blood pressure in a pregnant woman who is past 5 gestation months, careful observation should be made of the fetal heart tones.)
   D. Progressive drop in blood pressure and increase in pulse rate.
   E. Pain (e.g. substernal, in either shoulder and radiating down the arm or in the feet and legs).
   F. Changes in skin color (e.g. red, pale, bluish, mottled).
   G. Pounding heart, palpitations.

H. Difference between apical and radial pulse rates.
I. Edema (e.g. urticaria, dependent, generalized).
J. Extreme body temperature changes.
K. Extreme thirst.
L. Inappropriate fatigue.
M. Behavioral changes (e.g. apathy, apprehension, restlessness, irritability, confusion, delirium or disorientation).
N. Dizziness, visual changes, loss of consciousness.
O. Numbness, tingling of extremities.
P. Large, tortuous engorged veins.

3. A patient's blood pressure and pulse should be evaluated in relation to such factors as:
   A. His usual blood pressure and pulse.
   B. Age.
   C. Weight-height comparison.
   D. Posture.
   E. Physical activity.
   F. Emotional state.
   G. The diagnosed disease condition.
   H. Medications.
4. The pulse should be counted over whichever artery is most convenient and easy to palpate.
   A. When irregularities occur in the cardiac rhythm, a more accurate heart rate can be counted by listening to the apical heart beat with a stethoscope.
   B. When a cast has been applied and is drying, the pulse distal to the injury should be checked frequently (e.g. every 10 to 15 minutes).
5. When a blood pressure measurement cannot be made over the brachial artery, the ausculatory and/or palpatory methods may be used with other arteries (e.g. radial, popliteal, or dorsalis pedis arteries).
6. When the patient has injury to the brain (or possibility of injury), a rise in blood pressure and a fall in pulse should be reported immediately. The same is true if there is an ensuing fall in blood pressure accompanied by a rapid and weak pulse.
7. When local applications of heat or cold are made, the skin

should be observed closely for color change. Treatment should be discontinued if the color change is unusual (e.g. bright red, white, cyanotic) or persistent (e.g. more than 5 to 10 minutes).

8. When there is a possibility of a large quantity of blood pooling in the periphery and/or splanchnic region (e.g. following sympathectomy for hypertension, first post-operative ambulation or with a warm bath), the patient should be protected from a rapid fall in blood pressure by such means as:
   A. The use of elastic stockings or an abdominal binder.
   B. Encouraging gradual postural changes.
   C. The avoidance of high temperature of warm baths.
9. The rate of flow of intravenous fluids should generally be relatively slow (less than 60-80 drops/minute) when the patient:
   A. Is an infant or a child under the age of 12. (The rate should be ordered.)
   B. Is over the age of 55.
   C. Has a condition which affects his heart or arteries.
   D. Has a head injury.
10. Straining at stool should be prevented (See Nursing Care Related to "I.") and this is of particular importance when the patient has:
    A. An elevated blood pressure.
    B. An abnormal heart (e.g. a diseased heart or one with a congenital defect).
    C. Rectal-anal surgery.
    D. Hemorrhoids.
11. Inadequate arterial circulation to tissues should be prevented by avoiding prolonged pressure against blood vessels or peripheral nerves.
    A. Position changes should be made frequently and good body alignment should be maintained.
    B. Air-rings, special mattresses, cradles and footboards may be used.
    C. Restraints, tourniquets and blood pressure cuffs should be used with caution.

D. Close observation should be made of the circulation in an extremity when a cast, traction or any bandaging has been applied.

E. A newly-applied wet cast should be handled and positioned so as to prevent pressure against it which could cause changes in its shape (e.g. the cast should have a soft but firm and even support).

F. Umbilical cord prolapse should be prevented during labor by encouraging the pregnant woman whose membranes have ruptured to remain in a horizontal position. (This is particularly important when the presenting part is not engaged.)

G. When prolapse of the umbilical cord does occur, the pressure of the presenting part against the cord should be lessened (e.g. positioning, exertion of pressure against it), the doctor should be notified immediately and preparations should be made for an immediate Caesarian section.

12. Care should be taken to prevent anything which might cause the obstruction of a blood vessel from entering the general circulation.

A. Oily preparations should never be injected into the blood stream.

B. Care should be taken to prevent air from entering the blood stream during intravenous administrations of medications.

C. When there is a possibility of phlebothrombosis in an extremity the patient should be placed in a horizontal position, the affected part should be at rest and the symptoms reported promptly.

D. When tranfusions are ordered, arrangements should be made for typing and cross-matching to be done.

E. All blood used for transfusions should be positively identified before administration.

F. If a patient receiving a transfusion complains suddenly of sharp chest pains or chills and fever, the transfusion should be stopped and the symptoms reported immediately.

13. Normally, circulation to tissues may be increased by:
    A. Local application of heat or alternating heat and cold.
    B. Active or passive exercise.
    C. Massage.
14. Following delivery the uterus should be maintained in a contracted state by:
    A. Uterine massage.
    B. Preventing distention of the urinary bladder.
    C. Administration of oxytocic drugs as ordered.
15. When there is active bleeding or a danger of potential bleeding from injured blood vessels, muscular activity of or around the injured part (or possibly of the entire body) should be restricted.
16. When an observable source of bleeding has been determined,
    A. Direct pressure should be placed over the source whenever this is practicable.
       (Exceptions to this include bleeding from the ear or over the larynx.)
    B. A large artery supply to an injured extremity may be occluded by external pressure.
       (1) Pressure points may be used.
       (2) A tourniquet may be used with caution.
17. When bleeding occurs in an extremity, the affected part may be elevated above the heart.
    (An exception to this is when the need for immobilization supersedes the importance of stopping the bleeding.)
18. When there are signs of bleeding from the gastro-intestinal tract, food and fluids should be withheld until the doctor is notified and orders are obtained. (An exception to this is a relatively small amount of rectal bleeding.)
19. When there is bleeding from the urinary tract following bladder or prostatic surgery, bladder irrigations should be done as ordered.
20. Disturbance of any blood clot formation or further injury to already damaged tissue should be prevented by:
    A. Using caution in wound cleansing or removal of dressings.
    B. Avoiding the insertion of any object into an orifice from which bleeding is or recently has been occurring.

21. When there is interference with the normal clotting mechanisms, extreme caution should be taken to prevent any injury to blood vessels in any part of the body.
    A. Caution should be used in mouth and skin care.
    B. The bed or bed rails may be padded.
    C. The body should be handled very gently.
    D. If there is a choice between giving a medication orally or hypodermically, the oral route should be used.
22. When the pulse rate becomes abnormally fast or slow, any drug which might be responsible (e.g. heart stimulants or heart depressants) should be withheld prior to the prompt notification of the doctor.
23. If an abnormally rapid or slow pulse occurs in a fetus, the doctor should be notified immediately and preparations should be made for a rapid delivery either through the pelvis or by section.
24. When the blood pressure becomes abnormally high or low, any drug which may be responsible (e.g. vaso-constrictors or vaso-dilators) should be withheld prior to the prompt notification of the doctor.
25. When the patient's blood pressure and/or circulating blood volume are increased abnormally high (indicated by such observations as elevated blood pressure, flushing of skin, carotid throbbing, headache or visual disturbances),
    A. The head of the bed be elevated.
    B. Provision should be made for physical and emotional rest.
    C. The rate of flow of any intravenous infusion should be slowed.
    D. Sedatives or vaso-dilators may be administered as ordered.
    E. The patient should be observed closely for signs and symptoms of pulmonary edema (may include dyspnea, coughing, noisy breathing and apprehension), and if these signs and symptoms occur,
        (1) The head of the bed should be elevated.
        (2) Morphine sulfate (or other narcotic or narcotic-like drug) should be administered promptly as ordered.
        (3) Equipment for administering oxygen under pressure may be obtained and used as ordered.

(4) Equipment for reducing circulating blood volume may be obtained (e.g. three tourniquets, phlebotomy set).

26. When the patient's circulating blood volume and/or blood pressure are abnormally low (indicated by such observations as low blood pressure, decreased pulse pressure, weak rapid pulse, no pulse, pale and cold skin, cyanosis, extreme thirst, tinnitus, apprehension and loss of consciousness),
    A. The patient should be placed in a horizontal position.
    B. The rate of flow of any intravenous fluid should be increased (within limits).
    C. Preparation should be made for the administration of whole blood, plasma or other intravenous fluids.
    D. Preparation should be made for the administration of a vaso-constrictor drug as ordered.
    E. The patient should be kept comfortably warm (without use of any hot applications).
    F. The patient should be observed for urinary suppression.
    G. Record should be made of any possible allergic involvement.
    H. And heart arrest occurs,
       (1) Preparation should be made for an intracardial injection of epinephrine.
       (2) Preparation may be made for opening of chest cavity for heart massage or other stimulation.
    I. And this is due to uterine bleeding in a pregnant woman in advanced labor, preparation should be made for an immediate delivery.
    J. And this is due to uterine bleeding in a pregnant woman in early labor or late in pregnancy and not in labor, preparation should be made for a Caesarean section.
27. When there is tissue edema and/or loss of plasma proteins, the patient's fluid intake and output should be carefully measured. (Urinary output, and possibly specific gravity, may be checked and reported frequently when there is rapid loss of fluid and/or proteins.)
28. When the patient's condition warrants a decrease in the work load of the heart,

A. Provision should be made for more than usual sleep and rest.
B. Physical activity should be limited and spread out during waking hours.
C. Emotional excitement should be avoided.
D. Small, easily digested meals should be provided.

29. When a patient has impaired peripheral venous circulation,
    A. Peripheral venous return may be encouraged by:
        (1) Elevation of the extremity.
        (2) Passive or active exercise of the affected extremity.
        (3) The use of elastic stockings.
        (4) Avoidance of pressure against veins (e.g. positioning, proper clothing.)
    B. Caution should be taken to avoid injury to the affected part.
    C. The affected extremity should be observed closely for signs of ulceration.
30. When a patient has impaired peripheral arterial circulation,
    A. Exercise should be limited to prevent pain.
    B. Postural changes should be made which will allow for as much circulation as possible.
    C. The extremity should be protected from any mechanical injury or pressure (e.g. use of cradle on the bed, proper clothing).
    D. Extreme caution should be used in any application of heat or cold.
       (Such applications should not be used unless ordered by a physician.)
    E. A comfortable temperature for the affected extremity should be provided by appropriate environmental temperature and adequate coverings.
31. When a patient has a condition in which there is interference with the coronary circulation, increases in physical activity should be made slowly and gradually, and careful observation of the patient's total response to the activity should be made and reported.
32. Giving the correct dose of the correct drug is of greatest importance when the mode of administration is intravenous.

PRINCIPLES OF ANATOMY AND PHYSIOLOGY UNDERLYING THE NURSING CARE

A. The blood serves as a means of transport for substances to and from the cells, and the volume and pressure of circulating blood must be maintained within certain limits to provide for changing demands of the organs.

Facts Related to Blood Volume

1. Blood volume varies with the body weight and surface area. (In infants and children the blood volume is somewhat less per kilogram of body weight and per square meter of body surface than in adults.)
2. Blood volume may be affected by variations in fluid balance within the body (e.g. loss of plasma from the blood in severe burns).
3. The cardiovascular system is a closed system, and blood is not usually found outside of the system except as it is found in the uterus related to reproductive functions.
   A. Approximately 2 to 8 ounces of venous blood, mixed with mucus and endometrial tissue, are lost during a normal menstrual period. (Normally, menstrual blood does not clot.)
   B. A fetus is dependent for its life upon the blood of the mother circulating through the placenta.
   C. Labor may be accompanied by a loss of blood-tinged mucus from the cervix.
   D. A loss of more than 500 cc. of blood during a delivery is above normal.
   E. Following delivery there is a flow of uterine discharge from the vagina which may last one week to 6 weeks. (The flow is similar to a heavy menstrual period with the discharge changing from bloody to serous to mucous in type.)
   F. Following delivery involution of the uterus occurs.
      (1) The fundus of the uterus should be firm and well below the umbilicus immediately after delivery.
      (2) The fundus of the uterus normally returns into the

pelvis at a rate of approximately one-half inch a day, starting about the level of the umbilicus the first postpartum day.

4. The average-sized adult has about 5 to 6 liters of blood. (Rapid loss of more than 30 per cent of the total blood volume is usually incompatible with life.)
5. Many of the body organs have relatively large blood supplies or storage spaces for blood. (These organs include the spleen, liver, the pregnant and postpartum uterus—to six weeks—the kidneys, lungs, muscles, skin and thyroid gland.)
6. The amount of blood circulating to the body parts may be limited by:
   A. Venous stasis (especially in the vessels of the splanchnic region, the skin or the lower extremities).
   B. Internal obstruction within the blood vessels (e.g. vasospasms, vaso-constriction, thrombus or embolus).
      (1) A thrombus may occur as the result of injury to the intima of a blood vessel, a slowing of the blood stream or decreased coagulation time.
      (2) A thrombus may be dislodged by an active blood flow.
      (3) An embolus may be a blood clot, fat globule, air bubble, agglutinated blood cells or fragments broken off from diseased heart valves.
      (4) Agglutination and/or hemolysis of red blood cells may occur as a result of mixing incompatible blood groups. (This involves a type of antigen-antibody reaction in which the antigen is in the red blood cells and the antibody is in the serum.)
      (5) In transfusions, a recipient's serum can agglutinate the donor's cells.
         (a) Type A blood will agglutinate the cells of both Type B and Type AB.
         (b) Type B blood will agglutinate the cells of both Type A and Type AB.
         (c) Type AB blood will not agglutinate cells of any other type of blood because there is no antibody in the serum.

(d) Type O blood will not be agglutinated by any other type of blood because there is no antigen in the cells.

C. External pressure exerted against the blood vessel (e.g. from tumors or pressure applied on the body surface).

(1) Occlusion of blood vessels for the purpose of stopping bleeding may be accomplished by the application of pressure against relatively large blood vessels which lie over bone. These blood vessels include:

(a) The internal maxillary artery in front of the ear.

(b) The facial artery about an inch forward of the angle of the jaw.

(c) The subclavian artery behind the inner end of the clavicle against the first rib.

(d) The brachial artery on the inner aspect of the upper arm, about half way between the shoulder and the elbow.

(e) The femoral artery in the mid-groin over the innominate bone.

(2) The small blood vessels in the uterus are arranged between the smooth muscle fibers in such a way that the uterine muscle contractions can partially occlude these blood vessels.

(a) Smooth muscle of the uterus normally contracts with mechanical stimulation (e.g. massage of the fundus).

(b) Interference with uterine contractions may be caused by the upward pressure against the uterus from a full urinary bladder.

D. Injury to the peripheral nerves innervating the affected part.

E. Cardiac output.

7. Pain results when muscle tissue has inadequate circulation.
8. When cardiac muscle has insufficient circulation, irregularities in its contractions may result.
9. The color of the skin and mucous membrane are affected by the amount and kind of blood in the superficial blood vessels (e.g. pale, flushed or cyanotic).

10. A generalized decrease in circulating blood volume is accompanied initially by an increase in heart rate and vasoconstriction of the small blood vessels in the skin, mucous membrane and intestines. (If the volume decrease is prolonged, circulatory collapse may result, which involves heart failure and loss of tone in the smooth muscle of the arterial blood vessels.)
11. Either a marked increase or decrease in the blood supply to the brain can cause loss of consciousness.
12. Increased tissue activity normally results in a marked increase in the blood supply to the active tissue (e.g. the gastro-intestinal tract during digestion or the skeletal muscles during exercise).
13. The normal blood clotting mechanism helps to protect the body against blood loss.
    A. Essentially, injured thrombocytes and tissues release chemical substances which react with globulin factors in the plasma (in the presence of calcium ions) to produce thromboplastin. Thromboplastin allows prothrombin to become thrombin. The thrombin reacts with the fibrinogen in the serum to produce fibrin which forms the network of the clot.
        (1) The average platelet (thrombocyte) count is 250,000 per cu. mm. of blood.
        (2) Prothrombin and fibrinogen are produced in the liver.
        (Vitamin K, a fat-soluble vitamin produced by microbial action on certain kinds of food in the intestinal tract, is needed for the production of prothrombin.)
    B. Blood, after it is shed, normally clots within 3 to 5 minutes (clotting time).
    C. Bleeding from punctured skin capillaries normally ceases within 2 minutes (bleeding time).
    D. Prothrombin time measures the concentration of prothrombin in the blood. (When the amount is less than 10 per cent of the normal, there is a bleeding tendency; at 3 per cent, there is real danger.)

14. When there is bleeding high in the gastro-intestinal tract and blood is digested, the iron contained in the hemoglobin causes the feces to be black in color.

Facts Related to Blood Pressure

1. Arterial blood pressure can be defined as the amount of pressure exerted by the blood against the walls of the arterial blood vessels.
2. Arterial blood pressure varies with:
   A. The stroke-volume of the ventricular contractions.
      (1) The greater the force, the higher the pressure.
      (2) The greater the volume, the higher the pressure.
   B. The caliber of the arterioles. (The smaller the caliber, the higher the pressure.)
   C. The elasticity of the blood vessel walls. (The more rigid the walls, the higher the pressure.)
   D. The viscosity of the blood.
      (1) The greater the viscosity, the higher the pressure.
      (2) Blood is about 5 times more viscous than water.
3. Arterial blood pressure can be measured by equalizing external pressure applied against an artery with the pressure within the artery.
   A. Systolic pressure is the pressure at the time of ventricular systole.
      (1) The systolic measurement affords information about the cardiac output and the state of the peripheral blood vessels.
      (2) Taken in the brachial artery, the average range for an infant is 55 to 80 mm. of Hg. and the average range for an adult is 90 to 145 mm. of Hg.
   B. Diastolic blood pressure is the pressure at the time of ventricular diastole.
      (1) The diastolic measurement affords information about the basic pressure in the circulatory system.
      (2) Taken in the brachial artery, the average range for an infant is 40 to 50 mm. of Hg. and the average range for an adult is 60 to 90 mm. of Hg.

C. Arterial blood pressure can be determined in any extremity where a blood pressure cuff can be applied closely above a point where a pulse can be felt.

D. The blood pressures in opposite extremities may vary.

E. Visible strong pulsations of the carotid arteries indicates a high systolic pressure.

4. The pulse is the resultant throb in an artery caused by the rise and fall of the arterial pressure.

   A. The pulse can be felt wherever a superficial artery can be held against firm tissue.

   B. The strength of a pulse varies with the amount of systolic discharge and the elasticity of the arterial wall.

5. The pulse pressure is the difference between the systolic and diastolic pressures.

   A. The pulse pressure varies directly with the amount of blood ejected by the systolic discharges.

   B. The average range of pulse pressure is 30 to 50 mm. of Hg.

6. Postural changes affect arterial blood pressure.

   A. A sudden change from a lying position to a sitting or standing position can result in a sudden decrease in the supply of blood to the brain.

   B. There is an immediate rise in blood pressure when the position is changed from lying to sitting to standing.

7. Strenuous physical exercise (or contemplation of it) has the greatest of all physiological effects in raising the blood pressure. (The heavier the body, the greater is the amount of energy required for physical exercise.)

8. The amount of blood pumped from the ventricles into the arteries is determined by:

   A. The stroke-volume of the ventricular contractions.

   B. The integrity of the atrioventricular valves.

   C. The patency of the semilunar valves.

9. The amount of blood which reaches the ventricular chambers is determined by:

   A. The patency of the atrioventricular valves.

   B. The amount of venous return.

      (1) Venous return is determined, in part, by the rate of cardiac contractions.

(2) Venous return from the pulmonary circulation varies with the rate of blood flow through the pulmonary circuit and the volume and pressure of blood in the left side of the heart.

(3) Venous return from the systemic circulation varies directly with the gravitational force, the arterial blood pressure and the movement of the voluntary muscles and varies inversely with the intrathoracic pressure.

10. The work of the heart is dependent chiefly upon the amount of blood ejected per minute against the average pressure in the pulmonary or systemic circulation.
    A. The force of cardiac muscle contractions varies directly with the degree to which the ventricular chambers are filled with blood. (A rapid increase in the circulating blood volume markedly increases the work load of the heart.)
    B. The higher the blood pressure in the periphery and/or in the lungs, the greater is the force required by ventricular contractions to maintain an adequate blood flow. (A rise in the intra-abdominal pressure against the great vessels increases the systemic blood pressure.)
    C. Cardiac output is increased when there is an abnormal arterio-venous shunt in the heart or through the ductus arteriosus.
    D. Cardiac output is increased when body tissues require an increased amount of blood (e.g. skeletal muscles during exercise).
11. The heart muscle receives blood through the coronary circulation. (Following myocardial infarction, collateral circulation can be increased gradually and be successful in adequately supplying blood to the affected area.)
12. A compensated heart is one in which hypertrophy of cardiac fibers has increased the contractile power of the fibers so that the heart is able to attain some degree of normal function. (The degree of compensation will vary in individuals.)
13. In general, the heart rate bears an inverse relationship to:
    A. The size of the individual (e.g. the average rate for the

newborn is 130 to 140 beats per minute while the average rate for an adult at rest is 70 to 80 per minute).

B. The arterial blood pressure.

14. In general, the heart rate bears a direct relationship to the metabolic rate (e.g. an increased rate is seen during muscular exercise, digestion and in fever).
15. The heart rate may be accelerated or depressed by:
    A. Neural mechanisms.
       (1) The cardiac accelerator center is located in the medulla and operates through the thoraco-lumbar division of the autonomic nervous system.
       (2) The cardiac inhibitor center is located in the medulla and the vagus nerves carry inhibitory impulses to the sino-atrial node and sino-ventricular node.
    B. Hormonal influence.
       (Epinephrine causes an increased heart rate.)
16. The coordination of sequence in heart action—rhythmicity—is a function of the conduction system.
17. The apical heart beat can be heard best at the fifth intercostal space, slightly to the left of the sternum. (There are 2 sounds: the first is caused by the closing of the atrioventricular valves and the second is caused by the closing of the semilunar valves.)
18. The heart beats of a fetus can generally be heard by the fifth month of pregnancy. (The average rate of heart beats is 120 to 160 beats per minute.)
19. The walls of the arterioles contain smooth muscle which is under autonomic nervous control.
    A. Vaso-constriction results from sympathetic stimulation.
    B. Vaso-dilatation results from inhibition of the sympathetic stimulation.
    C. Blood pressure is greatly affected by the emotional state of an individual.
20. The vasomotor centers are located in the medulla.
21. Local vaso-dilatation may be caused by:
    A. The local application of heat.
    B. A temporary application of cold.
    C. Tissue injury.

D. Histamine or histamine-like substances.

22. Local vaso-constriction may be caused by:
    A. The local application of cold.
    B. Reflex mechanisms (e.g. vaso-constriction of the nasal and pharyngeal mucosal vessels when cold air is directed at the back or arms).
23. Generalized vaso-constriction may be caused by:
    A. Vasopressor substance produced in the posterior pituitary.
    B. Pressor principle called angiotonin (or hypertensin) which may be produced in the body as an indirect result of impaired kidney circulation.
    C. Nor-epinephrine.
24. Plasma contains all of the blood elements except the blood cells.
25. The cerebrospinal and intraocular fluids, formed from the blood, are absorbed continuously into the venous system. (Because there is a close relationship between the blood pressure and pressure of fluids in other closed fluid systems connected with the cardiovascular system, sudden blood pressure changes are reflected in the pressures of the cerebrospinal fluid and the intraocular fluids.)
26. A reduced arterial blood pressure, resulting in reduced renal flow causes decreased glomerular filtration in the kidneys. (A systolic pressure of more than 50 mm. of Hg. is needed for glomerular filtration.)
27. High blood pressure can cause rupture of a weakened arterial wall.
28. When the circulatory rate is slowed beyond certain limits,
    A. The veins may become engorged with blood containing reduced hemoglobin.
    B. The walls of the veins may become weakened (e.g. with resultant varicosities).
    C. The valves in the veins may become incompetent.
    D. Local or generalized edema may result.
29. The normal circulation rate of blood from one arm to the other or from one arm to the leg on the opposite side is about 20 seconds.

PRINCIPLES OF PHYSICS UNDERLYING THE NURSING CARE

A. The blood serves as a means of transport for substances to and from the cells and the volume and pressure of circulating blood must be maintained within certain limits to provide for changing demands of the organs.

1. Pressure is the force exerted on a unit area.
2. Fluids flow from an area of higher pressure to one of lower pressure, and the rate of volume flow is directly related to the pressure gradient.
3. The principle underlying liquid manometers, used for measuring pressures, is that the pressure beneath the free surface of a liquid is equal to the vertical height of the liquid times its density.
4. Gravitation is the force of attraction between two objects (e.g. the earth and an object on or near the earth).
5. Viscosity (fluid friction) is the internal resistance of fluid in motion and retards flow.

PRINCIPLES OF CHEMISTRY UNDERLYING THE NURSING CARE

A. The blood serves as a means of transport for substances to and from the cells and the volume and pressure of circulating blood must be maintained within certain limits to provide for changing demands of the organs.

1. Lipids are insoluble in water.
2. Plaster of Paris powder combines with water to form a solid mass of large crystals of gypsum, which occupy a larger volume than the original powder and water.
3. Some plastic materials used for casts shrink as they dry.

Section B: Nursing Care and Science Principles Related to Oxygen.

B. All the cells of the body require an adequate oxygen supply.

NURSING CARE

1. Patients should be observed for signs and symptoms of oxygen insufficiency, and these should be reported. This is of particular importance when the patient has:
   - A. Depression of the central nervous system (e.g. due to narcotics, anesthesia or inadequate circulation).
   - B. Injury—or possible injury—to medulla and/or cervical spinal cord or cervical nerves (e.g. in poliomyelitis, cervical fractures or pressure changes within the skull).
   - C. Injury to the lung tissue or pleura.
   - D. Irritation of the respiratory tract (e.g. by instruments, foreign bodies, micro-organisms or fumes).
   - E. Obstruction of the airway (e.g. in asthma, bronchitis, laryngeal edema or foreign body in airway).
   - F. Decrease in amount of lung tissue available for oxygen diffusion (e.g. in pneumonia).
   - G. Decrease in vital capacity (e.g. due to air or fluid in pleural cavity, inelasticity of lung tissue or pressure against diaphragm).
   - H. Impairment of circulation (e.g. in right-sided heart failure or congenital heart disease).
   - I. Anemia.
2. Reportable signs and symptoms of interference with adequate oxygen supply may include:

A. Abnormal breathing patterns.
  (1) Dyspnea.
  (2) Rapid, shallow breathing.
  (3) Different kinds of periodic breathing (e.g. Cheyne-Stokes).
  (4) Slow and/or very deep breathing (e.g. in acidosis).
  (5) Noisy breathing.

B. Skin color changes (e.g. cyanosis, extreme pallor), which may be most easily observable in the lips, around the mouth, and in the nailbeds.

C. Rapid, thready pulse, palpitations.

D. Coughing, choking, sneezing, singultus.

E. Apprehension, restlessness, sleeplessness.

F. Confusion, dizziness, loss of consciousness.

G. Irritability, headache.

H. Fatigue.

3. A respiratory rate can be counted most accurately if the patient is unaware of the procedure.
4. When central nervous system depressants are being administered (e.g. narcotics), respirations should be observed closely and any significant slowing of the rate should be reported promptly. (The depressant drug should be withheld until the doctor makes a decision about its continued use.)
5. Obstruction of the airway should be avoided by:

A. Preventing any oral intake of food or fluids
  (1) Several hours prior to the administration of a general anesthetic.
  (2) When the patient is unable to swallow.

B. Use of positioning.
  (1) Lying flat on side or abdomen with the head to the side and possibly lower than the trunk may be desirable.
  (2) Hyper-extension of the cervical spine should be avoided.
  (3) Frequent position changes of the unconscious patient, the patient who does not move himself, the patient who has had chest surgery and the elderly patient should be made.

C. Encouraging coughing when there may be excessive mucous production (e.g. following chest surgery).
D. Discouraging laughing or talking when there is anything solid or fluid in the mouth.
E. Use of an airway in an unconscious patient.
F. Keeping the mandible up and forward in an unconscious patient whose tongue has a tendency to fall backward.
G. Avoiding the entrance of any liquid into the respiratory tract which cannot be absorbed by the mucosa of the tract.
   (1) Nasal tubes should not be lubricated with oil.
   (2) The use of oily nose drops (not prescribed) should be discouraged.
   (3) Caution should be observed in the administration of nose drops and drugs which are given by inhalation.
   (4) Only *very* small amounts of physiological saline solution should be used in tracheotomy tubes when this treatment is ordered.
   (5) Gastric tubes should be inserted correctly and checked for proper placement.

6. When a patient has acute anoxia, nursing measures should be initiated immediately and a physician should be notified as indicated.
   A. If there is an obstruction in the airway, the obstruction should be removed as much as possible before using other methods to relieve anoxia.
      (1) Coughing may be encouraged.
      (2) The nares, pharynx, larynx and trachea may be suctioned.
      (3) The head may be lowered below the trunk.
      (4) Dentures may be removed.
      (5) Equipment may be prepared for a tracheotomy.
      (6) Epinephrine may be prepared for administration as ordered if there is bronchiolar constriction.
      (7) If asthmatic symptoms occur during the administration of a transfusion, the transfusion should be stopped.

B. If any obstruction has been removed as much as possible and insufficient oxygen is reaching the lung capillaries,
   (1) Oxygen may be administered.
   (2) Vital capacity may be increased by such methods as:
      (a) Elevating the head of the bed or placing the chest in a hyperextended posture.
      (b) Alleviating pain by use of medications, splinting of the chest and positioning.
      (c) Changing position so that the unaffected lung is allowed the greatest expansion possible.
      (d) Ascertaining that any drainage of fluid or air from the pleural cavity through tubes is adequate.
      (e) Covering securely any external opening into the pleural cavity.
      (f) Encouraging the use of abdominal muscles in expiration (e.g. in emphysema).
      (g) Encouraging the use of upper thoracic muscles in inspiration when the patient is in a body cast.

C. If the respiratory muscles are not functioning properly,
   (1) Artificial respirations may be used.
   (2) A respirator may be prepared (and used if ordered).
   (3) Respiratory stimulants may be prepared for administration as ordered.
   (4) The skin may be stimulated with rapid external temperature changes.
   (5) Breath may be exhaled directly into the mouth of the patient.
   (6) Rectal stimulation may be used.
   (7) A positive pressure apparatus for the administration of oxygen may be prepared and used as ordered.

7. When a patient has anoxia due to poor circulation or inadequate oxygenation of erythrocytes,
   A. Oxygen may be administered.
   B. Postural changes may be made as indicated (e.g. horizontal position).
   C. Some metabolic process may be slowed down by such methods as:

(1) Limiting exercise.
(2) Limiting digestive processes (e.g. by type and amount of diet).
(3) Eliminating excessive external stimuli.
(4) Providing for a comfortable body temperature.
(5) Avoiding emotional stress-producing situations.

8. When a patient has closed chest drainage or chest suction, great care should be taken to prevent the entrance of fluid or air into the chest (e.g. checking tubing connections, keeping bottles below the chest level or guarding against bottle breakage).
9. When a patient has irritation of the respiratory tract,
   A. He may be encouraged to avoid or to limit smoking, talking or laughing.
   B. Steam inhalations or other humidifiers may be helpful.
   C. The external temperature should be kept comfortably warm.
   D. Medications which act locally (e.g. cough syrups) or indirectly, through affecting the cough reflex, may be administered as ordered to relieve coughing.
10. When a patient is receiving mask oxygen over a prolonged period of time or is being given oxygen under pressure, he should be observed closely for symptoms of oxygen poisoning, and these should be reported. (Early symptoms may be substernal distress and disturbed cerebral activity.)
11. When a patient has singultus (hiccoughs), he may be encouraged to hold his breath briefly or to breathe in and out of a paper bag.
12. When a newborn premature infant receives oxygen for a prolonged time, the oxygen concentration should not exceed 40 per cent.
13. Extreme caution should be taken in administrating any preparation of carbon dioxide.

PRINCIPLES OF ANATOMY AND PHYSIOLOGY UNDERLYING THE NURSING CARE

B. All the cells of the body require an adequate oxygen supply.

Facts Related to Obtaining Oxygen from the External Environment

1. Oxygen can reach the alveoli of the lungs by passing through the nose and/or mouth, pharynx, larynx, trachea, bronchi and bronchioles.
2. There is no cartilage support in the respiratory tree below the terminal bronchioles.
3. The walls of the bronchioles contain smooth muscle which is under autonomic nerve control.
   A. Parasympathetic nerves cause bronchiolar constriction; sympathetic nerves allow for relaxation.
   B. Bronchiolar constriction may result from irritation of the sensory receptors in the mucosa of the upper respiratory tract.
4. Air and food have a common passageway through the pharynx.
   A. Normally, swallowing and breathing do not occur simultaneously.
   B. During swallowing, the larynx raises to meet the epiglottis and this closes off the laryngeal opening.
   C. Normally, pressure in the oropharynx causes swallowing.
5. If the muscles which protrude the tongue are put out of action (e.g. the result of paralysis or loss of consciousness), the tongue falls back against the pharynx. (Keeping the mandible up and pushed forward helps to prevent the tongue from falling backward.)
6. The respiratory tract is lined with epithelium which contains many mucus-secreting cells:
   A. Increased or decreased mucus production may occur when this membrane is irritated.
   B. The membrane is able to absorb *very* small amounts of aqueous solutions only.
7. Sneezing and coughing are protective reflexes concerned with

the expulsion of foreign material from the respiratory tract.

A. There are nerve centers in the medulla which are concerned with these functions.

B. The cough reflex may be initiated by stimulation of afferent nerve endings in the tracheal bifurcation, laryngeal mucosa, lung tissue or pleura by such factors as dryness, excessive fluid, foreign bodies, cold air, laughing, talking, smoke or other irritant fumes. (The nasal mucosa which has many superficial blood vessels helps to both moisten and warm inhaled air.)

C. The sneeze reflex may be initiated by stimulation of sensory receptors in the nasal or nasopharyngeal mucosa.

8. Air, containing oxygen, is caused to enter and leave the respiratory tract because of the intermittent periodic production of pressure changes in the intrapulmonic cavity.
   A. The mechanical process of breathing is accomplished by movements of the chest wall and diaphragm.
   B. During inspiration the diaphragm descends as it contracts and the rib cage is lifted upward and outward by:
      (1) The external intercostal muscles in quiet breathing.
      (2) The sternocleidomastoid muscles, the scalenes, the thoraco-humeral, and thoraco-scapular muscles in heavy breathing. (Relaxation of the abdominal muscles allows for a greater diaphragmatic contraction.)
   C. During expiration the diaphragm ascends as it relaxes and the rib cage is drawn downward and inward by:
      (1) The relaxation of the diaphragm and external intercostal muscles in quiet breathing.
      (2) The contraction of the internal intercostal muscles and abdominal muscles in heavy breathing.
9. Collapse of lung tissue is prevented by the maintenance of an intrapleural pressure which is less than atmospheric pressure.
10. Sub-atmospheric pressure changes in the intrapleural space cause similar changes in the intrapulmonic pressures.
11. Vital capacity is the total amount of air which can be exhaled after a maximal inspiration. Factors which affect vital capacity include:
    A. The structure of the chest wall.

B. The movement of the rib cage and diaphragm.
C. The elasticity of the lung tissue.
D. The amount of room available for lung expansion.

12. The average respiratory rate of a person at rest varies with age.
    A. The average rate for the newborn is 30 to 50 respirations per minute.
    B. The average rate for an adult is 16 to 20 respirations per minute.
13. A respiratory rate of less than 8 respirations per minute may fail to provide an adequate supply of oxygen, depending to some extent upon the depth of the respirations.
14. Because of the dead air space, shallow breathing can fail to supply sufficient oxygen.
15. The visceral and parietal pleura are serous membranes which are kept slightly moist by serous fluid.
    A. The serous fluid helps to prevent friction during the respiratory movements.
    B. When irritated, this membrane may produce increased or decreased amounts of serous fluids.

Facts Pertaining to the Nervous and Chemical Control of Respirations

1. The inspiratory and expiratory nerve centers are located in the medulla oblongata; the pneumotaxic, in the pons varolii. (The inspiratory center initiates inspiration; the expiratory, expiration; and the pneumotaxic acts as an inhibitor of inspiration.)
2. The internal and external intercostal muscles are innervated by spinal nerves arising from the thoracic spinal cord.
3. The auxiliary respiratory muscles are innervated by spinal nerves which arise at the cervical and thoracic levels of the spinal cord.
4. The phrenic nerve, which arises from the cervical level of the spinal cord, innervates the diaphragm.
5. Periodic spasms of the diaphragm (singultus) may be caused by abnormal stimulation of the respiratory centers or the diaphragm itself and can, over a prolonged time, markedly

affect breathing. (Increasing the carbon dioxide tension of the blood will sometimes stop the spasms.)

6. The nervous control of the rate and depth of respirations is influenced by chemical stimulation of the respiratory centers.
   A. Inspiring air containing over 3 per cent or less than 10 per cent carbon dioxide causes an increase in the rate and depth.
   B. Inspiring air which contains less than 0.4 per cent or more than 10 per cent carbon dioxide causes a decrease in rate and depth.
   C. A fall in the pH of the blood usually causes a temporary increase in rate and depth.
   D. Following an initial stimulation of respirations, oxygen lack depresses the respiratory centers.
7. Different types of periodic breathing indicate effects of various factors (e.g. pH of blood) upon the respiratory centers.
8. The respiratory rate and depth can be controlled to a limited extent by volition.

Facts Pertaining to the Transportation of Oxygen to the Cells

1. The diffusion of oxygen from the alveoli into the capillary blood is dependent upon such factors as:
   A. The amount of permeable membrane.
   B. Partial pressure gradients.
2. The respiratory part of the lungs receives its blood from the pulmonary arteries, the blood being returned via the pulmonary veins to the left side of the heart.
   A. Mixing of oxygenated and unoxygenated blood can occur in the heart if the foramen ovale is not closed.
   B. Mixing of oxygenated and unoxygenated blood can occur in the ascending aorta if the ductus arteriosus is not closed.
3. Most of the oxygen is carried to the body cells in combination with hemoglobin.
   A. The amount of oxygen which can be carried by a given volume of blood is dependent upon the amount of hemoglobin contained in the red blood cells in that volume of

blood. (Only very small amounts of oxygen can be dissolved in plasma.)

B. As a normal red blood cell matures, it loses its nucleus and is able to contain a larger amount of hemoglobin.
   (1) Erythroblasts and normoblasts are immature red blood cells and contain very little hemoglobin.
   (2) Extensive hemolysis, which may occur as a result of antigen-antibody reactions involving the red blood cells or in a disease such as malaria, usually causes severe chills and fever.

C. The normal red blood count for adults is about 4,500,000 to 5,000,000 per cubic millimeter of blood.

D. The normal range of hemoglobin is, in the adult, 12 to 15 grams per cent. (For the newborn infant these figures are slightly higher.)

E. The average volume of red blood cells following centrifuge is 40 per cent of the total volume.

F. The red blood cells of some individuals contain an antigen called the Rh factor which, when introduced into the blood of an individual without this antigen, causes the production of antibodies of the hemolytic type.

G. Oxygenated hemoglobin has a red color, while reduced hemoglobin has a bluish tinge.
   (1) An increase of reduced hemoglobin in the skin capillaries above 5 grams per cent generally gives the skin a bluish color and may indicate an insufficient oxygen supply.
   (2) Cyanosis is more clearly evident in regions where the skin is thin and unpigmented (e.g. lips, around mouth, nail beds).

H. Under normal conditions hemoglobin is 97 per cent saturated with oxygen in the lung capillaries. (Increasing the concentration of oxygen in the alveoli can cause a very slight increase in the amount of oxygen which will combine with hemoglobin.)

4. Carbon monoxide has a greater affinity for hemoglobin than does oxygen. (A high oxygen tension in the alveoli increases the rate of hemoglobin-carbon monoxide dissociation in the lung capillaries.)

Facts Pertaining to the Use of Oxygen by the Cells

1. The oxygen requirements of the cells vary directly with their metabolic rates. (Metabolic rates vary directly with the amount of thyroid hormone, the amount of cellular activity and the body temperature.)
2. Cellular metabolism varies directly with available oxygen.
   A. Abnormalities in cellular function occur if there is insufficient oxygen.
   B. Striated muscle can build up some oxygen debt, while nervous tissue and cardiac tissue cannot.
3. An individual can live only a few minutes without oxygen.
   A. The cells of the cerebral cortex may be damaged after as little as 30 seconds without oxygen and are generally irreparably damaged after as long at 5 minutes without oxygen.
   B. The cells of the brain stem are generally irreparably damaged after 25 to 30 minutes without oxygen.
   C. Anoxia usually causes anxiety with its associated symptoms (e.g. hyper-activity or sleeplessness).
4. An oxygen tension which is too high can inhibit enzyme activity, and thus have a poisoning effect on the body.
   A. Substernal distress is a primary symptom of oxygen poisoning.
   B. High concentrations of oxygen administered under pressure can cause convulsions.
   C. Prolonged exposure to high oxygen tension (over 40 to 50 per cent) with sudden transference to atmospheric oxygen can result in retinal damage in a new-born premature infant.

PRINCIPLES OF PHYSICS UNDERLYING THE NURSING CARE

B. All the cells of the body require an adequate oxygen supply.

1. Gravitation is the force of attraction between 2 objects (e.g. the earth and an object on or near the earth.)
2. Pressure is the force exterted on a unit area.

3. Fluids flow from an area of higher pressure to one of lower pressure.
   A. Differences between pressures are called pressure gradients. (The pressure of a given gas, even when it is mixed with other gases, depends upon its concentration alone.)
   B. The rate of volume flow is directly related to the pressure gradient.
4. Atmospheric pressure is the pressure exerted by the "sea of air" above the earth and is approximately 14.7 pounds per square inch or 760 millimeters of mercury at sea level.

PRINCIPLES OF CHEMISTRY UNDERLYING THE NURSING CARE

B. All of the cells of the body require an adequate oxygen supply.

1. Oxygen, carbon dioxide and carbon monoxide are all odorless and colorless gases.
2. The atmosphere at sea level contains approximately 20 per cent oxygen and 0.04 per cent carbon dioxide.
3. Under normal atmospheric pressure, most gases are only slightly soluble in water. (An increase in the pressure of a gas increases its solubility.)
4. The oxidation of carbon and hydrogen in foodstuffs by oxygen is an energy-liberating chemical reaction and when oxidation is complete, carbon dioxide and water are produced.
5. The size of the molecules allowed to pass through a permeable membrane depends upon the permeability of the membrane.
6. Physiological saline solution (isotonic with body fluids) is approximately a 0.9 per cent aqueous solution of sodium chloride.

Section C: Nursing Care and Science Principles Related to Nutrition.

C. All the cells of the body require adequate nutrition.

NURSING CARE

1. All patients should be observed for signs and symptoms of inadequate nutrition and these should be reported. This is of special importance when a patient has:
   A. A condition which affects the gastro-intestinal tract or the accessory structures.
   B. Psychic disturbances.
   C. A problem with food utilization (e.g. diabetes mellitus).
   D. Cancer.
   E. Chronic alcoholism.
2. Reportable signs and symptoms of inadequate nutrition may include:
   A. Abnormal change in weight.
   B. Weakness, fatigue, anorexia.
   C. Retarded growth, possibly mental retardation.
   D. Symptoms of hypoglycemia. (See Nursing Care Related to "G.")
   E. Symptoms of acidosis. (See Nursing Care Related to "F.")
   F. Symptoms of thyroid deficiency. (See Nursing Care Related to "G.")
   G. Symptoms of anemia. (See Nursing Care Related to "B.")
   H. Symptoms of electrolyte imbalance. (See Nursing Care Related to "E.")
   I. Bleeding tendency (e.g. ecchymosis, bleeding gums).
   J. Dry, hardened epithelial tissue.
   K. Night blindness.

L. Lesions of skin, tongue or mucous membranes.

M. Peripheral pain associated with muscles and joints.

N. Abnormal bone development (e.g. rickets) and abnormal conditions of teeth.

O. Excessive irritability.

P. Symptoms of jaundice. (See Nursing Care Related to "I.")

Q. Abnormal stools (e.g. diarrhea, containing much undigested foodstuffs or fatty stools).

3. A well-balanced diet includes adequate amounts of proteins, carbohydrates and fats and a choice of foods which provides adequate amounts of vitamins and minerals.

   A. When a well-balanced diet is not being eaten, recommendations may be made relative to the inclusion in the diet of foods which do provide adequate nutrients.

   B. Foods high in proteins and vitamins and minerals should be particularly encouraged when there is:
      (1) A rapid growth rate.
      (2) Pregnancy and lactation.
      (3) Healing or any development of new tissue (e.g. skin grafting).

   C. An increased caloric intake may be encouraged when there is:
      (1) Abnormally low weight.
      (2) A rapid growth rate.
      (3) An increased metabolic rate (e.g. in hyperthyroidism, fever).
      (4) Liver disease.
      (5) Lactation.

   D. A decreased caloric intake may be encouraged when reduction of weight is indicated.

   E. Food high in fat content may be discouraged when there is a condition involving:
      (1) The production, storage or availability of bile.
      (2) The inadequate production or availability of pancreatic juice.
      (3) Obesity.
      (4) Atherosclerosis.

F. Some exposure of the body to ultra-violet rays should be encouraged, especially in children.

4. All dietary orders should be followed specifically.
5. Appetite may be improved by:
   A. Providing a pleasant atmosphere.
      (1) Pleasant companionship may be helpful.
      (2) Unpleasant sights, noises or odors should be avoided.
   B. Providing for emotional and physical comfort.
      (1) Pain should be prevented or relieved.
      (2) Emotional disturbances should be prevented.
      (3) The mouth should be clean (e.g. in bronchiectasis, mouth care before meals is desirable).
   C. Providing for (as possible):
      (1) Attractive service of food.
      (2) Tasty food and variety of foods.
      (3) Foods which are particularly enjoyed and in keeping with cultural patterns.
      (4) Size of servings which are consistent with the individual's condition.
6. Eating may be encouraged by:
   A. Providing foods similar to usual diet.
   B. Providing foods which are at a desirable temperature.
   C. Providing for adequate understanding of the importance of eating.
   D. Providing for convenience of eating.
      (1) Food and utensils should be placed for convenience.
      (2) Food may be prepared for eating (e.g. breaking eggs or cutting meat).
      (3) A comfortable body position should be provided.
   E. Providing sufficient time for eating.
   F. Feeding or encouraging independence in self-feeding according to needs of each individual. (Tube-feeding may be done as ordered.)
7. Lactation may be encouraged by suckling of the infant and means may be provided for the emptying of the breast at each feeding.
8. Chewing food well before swallowing may be encouraged.

A. The condition of the mouth and teeth should be observed and abnormalities reported.

B. Tooth decay should be prevented by:

(1) Proper cleansing of the teeth.

(2) Encouraging good nutrition.

C. Adequate dentures should be provided as possible.

9. When chewing of food is not possible (e.g. due to absence of teeth) or the gastro-intestinal tract should have minimal stimulation, food should be finely chopped or in a liquid state.
10. Rest should be encouraged following meals.
11. Measures to prevent nausea, vomiting or regurgitation include:

A. Limiting physical activity (particularly after eating).

B. Avoiding motions conducive to nausea (e.g. turning from side to side).

C. Avoiding use of exaggerated Trendelenburg position within 2 to 3 hours after eating a meal.

D. Providing for position of greatest comfort.

E. Limiting amount of food or fluids taken and separating intake of solid foods and fluids. (A baby should be helped to bring up swallowed air frequently during and after feedings.)

F. Avoiding food when there is strong sympathetic stimulation (e.g. fear, emotional shock).

G. Discouraging oral intake of food or fluids as long as nausea or vomiting persists.

H. Giving food or fluids which would be least likely to cause gastric disturbance (e.g. bland, non-fatty diet, not excessively cold).

I. Avoiding the sensory stimulation of the uvula or posterior pharynx.

J. Avoiding use of eyes for fine work (e.g. reading).

K. Alleviating pain.

L. Providing for a pleasant environment with no strong stimuli (e.g. odors, sights or noises).

M. Recognizing emotional components and giving supportive care accordingly.

N. Administering anti-emetic or sedative drugs as ordered.
O. Reporting the symptoms.

12. Measures to prevent diarrhea include:
A. Limiting physical activity.
B. Providing for a pleasant environment with no strong stimuli (e.g. odors, sights or noises).
C. Discouraging oral intake of food or fluids which greatly stimulate intestinal peristalsis (e.g. raw fruits or vegetables).
D. Discouraging oral intake of food when increased peristalsis and diarrhea result.
E. Avoiding mechanical stimulation of the rectum (e.g. with thermometer).
F. Recognizing any emotional components and giving supportive care accordingly.
G. Administering anti-diarrheal or sedative drugs as ordered.
H. Reporting the symptom.

13. Symptoms of hypoglycemia may be relieved by eating foods rich in carbohydrate.

14. When there is a tube draining fluid from any part of the gastro-intestinal tract or from accessory structures,
A. The amount and type of drainage should be reported.
B. Abnormal amounts or types of drainage should be reported promptly.
C. The function of the tube should be maintained.
(1) The tubing and the amount of drainage should be checked frequently.
(2) The tube should be irrigated as ordered.
D. And it is ordered closed for a specified period of time and untoward symptoms occur (e.g. marked distention, severe pain, nausea, vomiting), the tube may be opened for drainage and this should be reported.
E. And it is removed (not ordered) or becomes dislodged, this should be reported promptly. (When a patient has had gastric surgery recently—within days—a removed or dislodged gastric or intestinal tube should not be replaced without a specific medical order to do so.)

15. Descriptions of vomiting should be reported in terms of:

A. Characteristics of the vomitus.
   (1) Amount.
   (2) Color.
   (3) Consistency.
   (4) Any unusual odor.
B. Characteristics of the vomiting.
   (1) Frequency.
   (2) Relation to ingestion of food.
   (3) Type (e.g. projectile or regurgitation).

16. The excessive and/or continued intake of nonabsorbable oil (e.g. mineral oil) without medical orders should be discouraged.

PRINCIPLES OF ANATOMY AND PHYSIOLOGY UNDERLYING THE NURSING CARE

C. All the cells of the body require adequate nutrition.

Facts Pertaining to the Gastro-Intestinal Tract in General

1. The digestive system prepares food for absorption, moves food along the tract and provides for the absorption of food into the blood and/or lymph.
2. The parts of the gastro-intestinal tract primarily concerned with digestion, movement of food along the tract and absorption are:
   A. The mouth.
   B. The esophagus.
   C. The stomach.
   D. The small intestines.
   E. The accessory structures, including:
      (1) The teeth.
      (2) The tongue.
      (3) The salivary glands.
      (4) The liver and gall bladder.
      (5) The pancreas.
3. In the process of mastication food is broken down into smaller pieces which can be acted upon more easily by enzymes.

A. The teeth, saliva and tongue are important in mastication.
B. Chewing involves both up and down and lateral movements of the mandible. (The muscles of mastication originate on the zygomatic arch or the skull and insert on the mandible.)
C. There are 3 types of teeth:
   (1) The incisors and canines, which are designed for biting.
   (2) The molars, which are adapted for grinding.
D. The teeth appear in 2 sets; first the deciduous, and later the permanent teeth.
   (1) There are 20 deciduous teeth which begin to erupt by the 6th to 9th month and are usually all erupted by the end of the 2nd year.
   (2) At about the 6th year, the 32 permanent teeth begin to erupt and usually all the permanent teeth have erupted by the 18th year.
   (3) Dentine is the exquisitely sensitive yellowish basis of the tooth.
   (4) Enamel is the white insensitive covering of the crown of the tooth. (Enamel, although the hardest substance in the body, can be decayed by the prolonged action of various acids upon it. An example is acid produced by the action of lactobacilli on food particles in the mouth.)
   (5) Pulp is fibrous material projecting up into the dentine and contains nerves and blood vessels.
G. There are 3 pairs of salivary glands, all of which have ducts which open into the mouth. (The parotid glands lie below and in front of the ears.)
H. The tongue is a muscular organ innervated by the hypoglossal nerve.

4. Food reaches the stomach through the esophagus.
   A. Saliva, produced by the salivary glands, aids in swallowing.
   B. Swallowing is accomplished by voluntary and involuntary actions.
      (1) The tongue pushes food back to the pharynx.

(2) When food reaches the posterior pharynx, it is carried to the stomach by both gravity and the peristaltic movements of the esophagus.

(3) There is a deglutition center in the medulla.

C. The cardiac valve is a sphincter muscle located between the esophagus and stomach.

(1) Pressure against the cardiac sphincter from stomach contents may cause regurgitation of foods.

(2) Spasm of the cardiac valve may be caused by overstimulation of the autonomic nerves which innervate it.

5. Gastric movements result in the mixing of food with the gastric juices and also cause the food to become semi-fluid, which provides for more thorough enzymatic action in the small intestines.

(Gastric motility is first increased by distention, then decreased.)

6. Food passes from the stomach to the duodenum through the pyloric sphincter.

A. The rate at which food passes through the pyloric sphincter varies with:

(1) The size of the opening.

(2) Gastric motility.

(3) The type of food. (Carbohydrates pass through most rapidly, protein next; fatty foods take the longest time.)

(4) The consistency of the food. (The more liquid the food, the faster it passes through.)

B. The stomach is emptied in 3½ to 4 hours after a normal-sized, mixed meal.

7. Peristaltic movements cause the chyme to pass through the duodenum, to the jejunum, to the ileum.

A. The rate of the passage varies with:

(1) The motility of the tract.

(2) The opening of the ileocecal valve. (Emotional excitement and swallowing of food increase the rate of opening.)

   B. The time of digestion in the small intestine usually does not exceed 2 to 4 hours.
8. The motility of the smooth muscle of the gastro-intestinal tract is:
   A. Increased by parasympathetic stimulation (e.g. in some emotional states).
   B. Decreased by sympathetic stimulation (e.g. in some emotional states).
   C. Generally increased by irritation of the mucosa of the tract.
   D. Affected by some drugs (e.g. laxatives, opiates or posterior pituitary hormone).
9. The amount of gastric juices secreted daily varies greatly but, under normal conditions, is usually about 2 to 3 liters in 24 hours. (The gastric juices are watery, clear and slightly yellow in color or colorless.)
10. The amount of intestinal digestive juices secreted daily varies greatly, but under normal conditions may be about 2 to 3 liters in 24 hours.
11. During digestion and absorption circulation in the digestive tract is increased.
12. Hunger occurs when:
    A. The stomach is empty and contracting.
    B. There is hypoglycemia.
13. Appetite and salivary and gastric secretion are affected by:
    A. An individual's emotional state.
       (1) Pleasant stimuli tend to increase them.
       (2) Unpleasant stimuli tend to decrease them.
    B. Stimulation of the gustatory end-organs.
14. Chemical or mechanical irritation of sensory receptors in the buccal or gastric mucosa generally causes increased salivation.
15. Gagging, vomiting and hypermotility of the intestinal tract are protective reflexes concerned with the expulsion of injurious material from the gastro-intestinal tract.
    A. Mechanical stimulation of the pharynx or uvula causes gagging which may result in vomiting.

B. Vomiting is accomplished primarily by the actions of the muscles of the abdominal wall.

C. The vomiting center, located in the medulla, may be affected by:
   (1) Afferent impulses from the stomach.
   (2) Strong sensations (e.g. taste, smell, pain or strong affectual reactions such as rage).
   (3) Afferent impulses from parts of the body concerned with equilibrium (e.g. eyes, cochlea or cerebellum).
   (4) Pressure on the center itself.
   (5) Some drugs.

D. Projectile vomiting is sudden, forceful vomiting which is not preceded by nausea or retching. (This type of vomiting is sometimes associated with increased intracranial pressure.)

Facts Pertaining to Food, Digestion and Metabolism in General

1. A food is any substance which when absorbed into the blood stream, may be used for:
   A. Building or repair of tissue.
   B. Synthesizing essential compounds (enzymes and hormones).
   C. Furnishing energy.
2. Adequate nutrition includes sufficient amounts of carbohydrates, fats, proteins, vitamins and minerals.
3. Digestion is the breaking down of foods (mechanical and chemical) prior to their absorption into the blood or lymph.
4. Metabolism is the sum of all the chemical reactions which occur in the body.

Facts Pertaining to Milk Production

1. Following parturition the mammary glands produce milk.
   A. Milk is produced from substances in the mother's blood.
   B. Two to 3 days following the birth of a child, colostrum is

produced. (Colostrum is thick yellowish fluid rich in protein and salts.)

C. After this, there is a gradual change in the mammary secretion until, by about 10 days, the product is milk.

2. The amount of milk produced varies with individuals, but may be as much as 1000 cc. within a 24-hour period.
3. Suckling of an infant and emptying of the breasts generally stimulates milk production.

Facts Pertaining to Carbohydrates

1. Carbohydrates are used mainly as a source of energy but are found in all protoplasm and in many important compounds of the body. (Each gram of carbohydrate yields four calories.)
2. Starch is the most abundant source of carbohydrate in the diet.
3. Carbohydrates must be hydrolyzed to monosaccharides before they can be absorbed.
4. The hydrolysis of carbohydrates is accomplished by the activity of several enzymes. (Most of the hydrolysis of carbohydrates is accomplished by enzymes in the pancreatic juice and intestinal juice.)
5. Monosaccharides are absorbed primarily in the small intestine.
6. Most of the glucose in the body is converted to glycogen before use, although glucose may be used directly without this conversion.
7. Excess amounts of glucose may be:
   A. Excreted through the kidneys (if the blood level is above 160-180 mg. per cent).
   B. Stored as glycogen in the liver and muscles.
   C. Converted to and stored as fat.
8. The non-nitrogen part of some of the amino acids is converted to glucose in the body.
9. The glycerol of fats may be converted to glucose in the body.
10. The liver plays an important role in the metabolism of carbohydrates.

Facts Pertaining to Lipids

1. Some of the fatty acids are essential constituents of protoplasm.
   A. Brain and nervous tissue are rich in lipids.
   B. Cholesterol is found in all cells.
   C. Lipids are important constituents of cellular membranes.
2. Fat provides the main store of reserve food supply. (Each gram of fat yields 9 calories.)
3. The digestion of lipids is accomplished by:
   A. The emulsification of fats by bile salts.
   B. The hydrolysis of fats, primarily by pancreatic lipase.
4. Bile is constantly secreted by the liver; it is stored and concentrated in the gall bladder.
   A. The presence of fat in the duodenum causes the contraction of the gall bladder.
   B. Bile is dark greenish-brown in color when it is exposed to air.
5. Fatty acids combine with bile salts for absorption into the lacteals in the villi of the ileum.
6. Both fatty acids and molecules of fat are utilized by the body.
7. When bile cannot pass into the duodenum through the common bile duct (or hepatic), it is absorbed into the circulatory system and jaundice results.
8. The liver plays an important role in fat metabolism.
9. Some oily substances are not hydrolyzed and cannot be absorbed (e.g. mineral oil), so pass through the gastro-intestinal tract and are eliminated with the feces. (The presence of such non-digested oils in the intestinal tract interferes with the absorption of fat-soluble vitamins.)

Facts Pertaining to Protein

1. There is a constant need for protein to build and repair tissue.
   A. The body does not store protein to any extent.
   B. The need for protein is relatively greater when growth is occurring.

C. The state of protein nutrition is an important factor in general health.

2. Protein not used for tissue building can be oxidized for energy. (Each gram of protein yields 4 calories.)
3. The hydrolysis of proteins into amino acids is accomplished by the action of enzymes.
   A. Pepsin in the stomach starts hydrolysis.
   B. Proteolytic enzymes in the pancreatic juice and the intestinal juice complete the hydrolysis.
4. Amino acids are absorbed through the villi of the small intestine and are the forms of protein utilized by the body.
5. Essential amino acids are those which the body is unable to synthesize.
6. The liver plays an important role in the metabolism of protein. (Urea, a waste product, is formed through the breakdown of amino acids, primarily by the liver.)

Facts Pertaining to Minerals

1. The following minerals are important to efficient cellular functioning:
   A. Calcium (bones and muscles).
   B. Phosphorus (bones, metabolism of glucose).
   C. Sodium (extracellular fluid).
   D. Potassium (intracellular fluid).
   E. Iodine (thyroid hormone).
   F. Iron (hemoglobin).
   G. Chlorides (extracellular fluid).
   H. Traces of others which are obtained in a well-balanced diet.
2. Vitamin D is essential to the normal absorption and metabolism of calcium.

Facts Pertaining to Vitamins

1. Vitamins are chemical substances which, if lacking in the diet, manifest their absence by certain disease conditions or abnormal body functions.
2. Vitamins A, D, E and K are fat-soluble. (Absorbable lipids

and bile salts are essential for these vitamins to be absorbed.)

3. A deficiency of Vitamin A results in dry, hardened epithelial tissues (e.g. of the skin, lining of the respiratory tract or eyes) and night blindness (because of Vitamin A's relationship to visual purple).
4. A deficiency in Vitamin D results in the improper calcification of bones. (Ergosterol in the body, obtained from the diet, plus ultra-violet rays on the skin results in the formation of Vitamin D.)
5. A deficiency in Vitamin K results in inadequate formation of prothrombin.
6. A deficiency in Vitamin C results in capillary fragility, loss of intercellular substance (especially in bones and teeth) and poor wound healing.
7. There are several fractions of Vitamin B.
   A. A deficiency in thiamin results in anorexia and polyneuritis.
   B. A deficiency in riboflavin results in lesions of the mouth, tongue and mucous membranes.
   C. A deficiency in niacin results in skin lesions and inflammation of the gastro-intestinal tract.
   D. A deficiency in pyridoxine results in nervousness and weakness.
   E. A deficiency in B-12 gives rise to immature red blood cells.
8. Some of the vitamins are essential for the structure of certain of the tissue enzymes.

PRINCIPLES OF PHYSICS UNDERLYING THE NURSING CARE

C. All the cells of the body require adequate nutrition.

1. Energy possessed by an object is the ability or capacity to do work. (Heat is a form of energy.)
2. A Calorie is the amount of heat needed to raise the temperature of one liter of water one degree Centigrade.
3. Surface tension of a liquid is the measurement of the tendency of a liquid surface to contract to the smallest possible area.

PRINCIPLES OF CHEMISTRY UNDERLYING THE NURSING CARE

C. All the cells of the body require adequate nutrition.

1. Surface tension of water may be decreased by bile salts.
2. The lowering of surface tension aids in the emulsification of lipids. (An emulsion is the colloidal suspension of one liquid in another.)
3. A catalyst is a substance which speeds a chemical reaction, but does not change permanently itself in the reaction.
4. The hydrolysis of a chemical substance is a process whereby a substance is broken down into simpler substances by reaction with water.
5. Starch is a polysaccharide which can be hydrolyzed to the disaccharide, maltose.
6. Maltose, sucrose and lactose are disaccharides which can be hydrolyzed to monosaccharides.
   A. Maltose is hydrolyzed to glucose.
   B. Sucrose is hydrolyzed to glucose and fructose.
   C. Lactose is hydrolyzed to glucose and galactose.
7. Lipids are esters of fatty acids and glycerol or other alcohols and simple lipids can be hydrolyzed to fatty acids and alcohols.
   A. Simple lipids include fats, oils, waxes.
   B. Compound lipids include phospholipids and glycolipids.
   C. Lipids are insoluble in water.
   D. Mineral oil is a hydrocarbon, not a lipid, and is not digestible. (Mineral oil will absorb fat-soluble vitamins.)
8. Proteins are very complex molecules, always containing nitrogen, and may be hydrolyzed to polypeptides, peptones, and finally to amino acids.

Section D: Nursing Care and Science Principles Related to Fluid Balance.

D. Definite amounts of water are essential to maintain the fluid balance of the body.

NURSING CARE

1. All patients should be observed for signs and symptoms of fluid imbalance (dehydration and edema) and these should be reported. This is of particular importance when the patient:
   A. Has a condition causing loss of fluid (e.g. burns, surgery, hemorrhage, diabetic coma, diarrhea or vomiting).
   B. Has a condition in which there is a slowing of circulation (e.g. heart failure or shock).
   C. Has a disease condition involving the pituitary gland, the thyroid gland or the adrenal cortex.
   D. Is receiving thyroid hormone, adrenal cortical hormones or adrenocorticotrophic hormone.
   E. Has a condition in which the plasma proteins, particularly albumen, are decreased (e.g. in liver disease).
   F. Has a urological condition.
   G. Is receiving diuretics or large quantities of fluids.
   H. Is pregnant.
2. Reportable signs and symptoms of fluid imbalance include:
   A. Signs and symptoms of dehydration, which may include:
      (1) Thirst.
      (2) Dryness of the skin and mucous membranes.
      (3) Fever.
      (4) Increased pulse rate.
      (5) Oliguria and highly concentrated urine.

(6) Constipation.
(7) Loss of weight.
(8) Exhaustion and collapse.

B. Signs and symptoms of fluid retention, which may include:
(1) Sudden weight gain.
(2) Puffiness of face, hands.
(3) Swelling of ankles, legs, feet.
(4) Abdominal distention.
(5) Headache, confusion, convulsions, coma.
(6) Dyspnea.

3. Measurement of fluid intake (all channels) and fluid output (all channels) should be made when:
A. The patient has a potential fluid imbalance (e.g. kidney disease or following major surgery).
B. The patient is suspected of having fluid imbalance.
4. When a patient has a tube draining fluid from the body into a container, the drainage should be measured.
5. Estimative descriptions should be reported of abnormal amounts of fluid lost;
A. From the skin (sweat or tissue fluid).
B. Through the gastro-intestinal tract (e.g. diarrhea or ileostomy).
C. On dressings.
6. When the average hourly urine output is less than 25 cc. or more than 500 cc., this should be reported promptly.
7. When urinary specific gravities are ordered, medical orders should be sought concerning the maximum or minimum values which should be reported promptly.
8. Polyuria, frequency and, possibly, involuntary micturition
A. Should be reported.
B. May be expected and should be provided for when the patient:
(1) Is cold.
(2) Is emotionally upset.
(3) Is unable to control the external urethral sphincter (e.g. in infancy or in motor nerve damage).
(4) Has diabetes mellitus (uncontrolled).

(5) Has hypoactivity of the posterior pituitary gland.
(6) Is receiving diuretics or large amounts of fluids.
(7) Is in first or third trimester of pregnancy.
(8) Has inflammation of the lower urinary tract or pelvic area.
(9) Has a cystocele.

9. Medical orders concerned with fluid intake or output should be sought when there is a potential problem of fluid imbalance.
10. Unless nausea and vomiting are occurring or it is ordered otherwise, oral fluids should be encouraged:
    A. When there is a problem of dehydration.
    B. When there is a systemic or urinary infection.
    C. When there is a problem (actual or potential) of urinary tract calculi.
    D. When the patient is receiving diuretics or sulfa drugs.
    E. During pregnancy and lactation.
11. The external environmental temperature should be controlled to prevent any preventable loss of fluid through sweating.
12. When there is a problem of edema,
    A. A daily weight may be taken (depending upon the patient's general condition).
    B. The sodium intake may be restricted.
    C. Care should be taken to avoid injecting medications into edematous tissue.
    D. Care should be taken to encourage as good a circulation as possible to parts of the body which are edematous (e.g. avoidance of pressure areas).
13. When fluid intake is to be restricted or to be forced, plans should be made for a reasonable distribution of fluids throughout the patient's waking hours.
14. Patients should be observed for signs and symptoms of a distended bladder (e.g. restlessness, pain, frequent voiding of small amounts, palpable bladder) and these should be reported. This is of particular importance when there is:
    A. Surgery involving the urological or reproductive tracts.
    B. Sensory and/or motor paralysis involving the bladder.

C. Problem of urinary obstruction (e.g. prostatic hypertrophy or plugged catheter).

15. A patient may be helped to empty his bladder by:
    A. Relieving or preventing embarrassment or tension.
    B. Helping him to assume as usual a position as possible for emptying the bladder.
    C. Listening to running water, putting his hands in water, having water poured over the genitalia, or sitting in a tub of warm water.
    D. Performing catheterizations as ordered.
16. A distended bladder should be emptied slowly.
17. The function of a tube for bladder drainage should be maintained by:
    A. Preventing kinking of the tubing.
    B. Preventing pressure against the tubing.
    C. Irrigating the catheter as ordered.

PRINCIPLES OF ANATOMY AND PHYSIOLOGY UNDERLYING THE NURSING CARE

D. Definite amounts of water are essential to maintain the fluid balance of the body.

Facts Pertaining to Fluid Balance in General

1. Diffusion, dialysis and osmosis are important processes underlying the interchange of materials between the cells and their surroundings, the regulation of blood volume and kidney function.
2. About 70 per cent of the body weight is water, 20 per cent of which is the extracellular fluid.
3. Normally, the body's fluid output balances the intake except when new tissues or fluids are being formed (e.g. during growth), and then fluid is retained.
4. The isotonicity of body fluids is maintained largely by the retention or elimination of water and certain electrolytes (sodium and potassium primarily) and is regulated by kidney function.
    A. A loss of sodium is followed by loss of water.
    B. The ingestion of sodium is followed by water retention.

C. The state of hydration of cells depends primarily upon the concentration of sodium ions in the extracellular fluid.

5. The amount of tissue fluid varies with:
   A. The filtration rate of fluid from the capillaries which varies, in turn, with:
      (1) The rate of blood flow (an inverse relationship).
      (2) The capillary blood pressure (a direct relationship).
      (3) The osmotic pressure of the blood (an inverse relationship).
      (4) The capillary dilatation (a direct relationship).
      (5) The concentration of sodium and proteins in the tissue fluid (a direct relationship).
      (6) The concentration of oxygen in the blood (an inverse relationship).
   B. The return of fluid from the intercellular spaces into the blood which varies, in turn, with:
      (1) The patency of the lymph channels (a direct relationship).
      (2) The pressure of the lymphatic fluid (an inverse relationship).
      (3) The concentration of sodium and proteins in the plasma (an inverse relationship).
      (4) The rate of blood flow (a direct relationship).
6. The plasma proteins, albumen and globulin, serve to maintain the osmotic pressure of the blood.
   A. These proteins are produced mainly in the liver.
   B. Albumen exerts the greatest force.
   C. The kidney glomerulus normally allows very little protein to pass into the tubule.
   D. Because albumen has the smallest molecular weight, it is the first protein to be able to pass through an injured kidney glomerulus.
   E. The normal serum protein is between 6 to 8 grams per cent.
   F. The normal A/G ratio is 1.5:1 to 3:1.
7. Edema is the excessive accumulation of fluids in the tissue spaces. It may occur in:

A. Areas of the body where connective tissue is particularly loose (e.g. face, hands or external genitalia).
B. The abdominal cavity.
C. The lungs.
D. The brain.
E. Dependent parts of the body (e.g. the feet when standing).
F. Small localized areas as part of the inflammatory process.

8. An excessive amount of tissue fluid interferes with the adequate exchange of substances between the cells and the blood.
9. Normally, when the fluid output exceeds the fluid intake, dehydration results.
   A. A loss of one fourth of the body water is usually fatal.
   B. Dehydration may be accompanied by:
      (1) Dryness of the skin and mucous membranes.
      (2) Thirst.
      (3) Elevated body temperature.
      (4) Increased pulse rate.
      (5) Loss of weight.
      (6) Exhaustion and collapse.
10. No appreciable amounts of tissue fluid are lost through the skin because of the continuous layers of keratinized epithelium.

Facts Pertaining to Fluid Intake

1. Thirst gives some indication of the amount of fluid intake needed.
2. Water may be replenished in the body by:
   A. Ingestion and absorption of food and fluids. (Absorption of water is a function of the colon.)
   B. Parenteral administration of fluids.
3. A healthy adult requires about 2500 cc. of water intake in a 24-hour period.

Facts Pertaining to Fluid Output

1. Water is lost from the body through the lungs, skin, kidneys and gastro-intestinal tract.

A. The average adult involved in a light occupation in a temperate climate loses daily approximately:
   (1) 1000 cc. of water from the skin (500 cc. of sweat and 500 cc. of insensible perspiration).
   (2) 1500 cc. of water from the kidneys.
   (3) 300 cc. of water from the lungs.
   (4) 150 cc. of water in the feces.

B. The amount lost through the kidneys varies inversely with the amount lost through other routes.

C. When the air is hot or the body temperature is elevated, the loss of water through the skin is increased.

2. The kidneys secrete urine continuously at the average rate of 60 to 120 cc. an hour. (Variations from 25 cc. to 500 cc. an hour may be considered to be within safe limits.)
3. A definite amount of water is necessary for the excretion of nitrogenous waste products by the kidneys and for maintaining in solution various threshold substances (e.g. calcium).
4. The volume of urine secreted varies with the amount of glomerular filtration and the amount of tubular reabsorption.

A. The amount of glomerular filtration varies directly with:
   (1) The amount of filtering surface.
   (2) The blood pressure in the glomeruli.
   (3) The amount of renal blood flow.
   (4) The rate of tubular absorption.

B. The amount of glomerular filtration varies inversely with the osmotic pressure exerted by plasma proteins.

C. The amount of tubular reabsorption of water varies directly with:
   (1) The water content of the blood.
   (2) The amount of anti-diuretic factor produced in the posterior pituitary.
   (3) The amount of adrenal cortical hormone secreted (because of the effect of sodium loss and potassium retention).
   (4) The blood level of estrogens.

D. The amount of tubular reabsorption varies inversely with:
   (1) The rate of blood flow in the efferent capillaries.

(2) The concentration of threshold substances in the tubules (e.g. glucose).

5. Urine volume is influenced by:
   A. Fluid intake (a direct relationship).
   B. Environmental temperature (an inverse relationship).
   C. Emotional stress (may be either direct or inverse relationship).
   D. Pain (inverse relationship).
   E. Age (an inverse relationship). (Infants excrete, for their weight, 3 to 4 times more urine than adults.)
   F. Diuretics (a direct relationship).
6. The average range of specific gravity is 1.010 to 1.030.
   A. The specific gravity varies inversely with the volume. (An exception to this occurs in uncontrolled diabetes mellitus when there is a high specific gravity and large amounts of urine.)
   B. Decreased fluid intake results in a concentrated urine.
7. Urine, freshly voided, is usually pale yellow to light amber in color and clear with no sediment.
   A. Urine which stands over a prolonged period of time normally develops a small amount of sediment.
   B. Urine which is highly alkaline (e.g. due to diet) is cloudy in nature.
   C. Freshly voided urine does not normally have an unpleasant odor.

Facts Pertaining to Elimination of Urine

1. Urine passes from the kidney pelvis through the ureters to the bladder where it is stored until released by reflex or voluntary action.
   A. Awareness of the need to void normally occurs when the bladder contains 300 to 500 cc. of urine. (The desire to void may be increased markedly when external pressure is exerted on the bladder or when the bladder or urethra is irritated.)
   B. A distended bladder can be palpated above the symphysis

pubis. (An adult bladder can hold up to 3000 to 4000 cc. of urine.)

C. The bladder wall contains sensory receptors which respond to the rise in pressure exerted on them as the bladder fills.

D. Continued stretch of the bladder wall produced by the accumulation of urine causes loss of bladder tone. (Recovery of the tone may occur more readily if the internal pressure is decreased gradually.)

E. The act of micturition involves the action of the detrusor reflex and the opening and closing of the sphincters.

   (1) The spinal reflex responsible for detrusor contraction can be inhibited or facilitated by nerve impulses from the higher centers.

   (2) The external sphincter can be powerfully closed by voluntary muscle contraction even when the detrusor contracts.

   (3) Involuntary micturition may occur as a result of emotional stress.

F. An overflow of urine from the bladder may occur when the pressure caused by the accumulation of urine is sufficient to overcome the normal tone of the sphincters and dribbling will continue until the pressure has been decreased enough for sphincter control to be resumed.

G. Weakness of the vaginal wall may result in the pouching of the bladder toward the vaginal orifice.

PRINCIPLES OF PHYSICS UNDERLYING THE NURSING CARE

D. Definite amounts of water are essential to maintain the fluid balance of the body.

1. Gravitation is the force of attraction between 2 objects (e.g. the earth and an object on or near the earth.)
2. Pressure is the force exerted on a unit area.
3. Fluids flow from an area of higher pressure to one of lower pressure and the rate of volume flow is directly related to the pressure gradient.

4. Specific gravity is the weight of an object compared with the weight of an equal volume of water. (Specific gravity can be determined by dividing the weight of 1.0 cc. of fluid by the weight of 1.0 cc. of water—which is 1.0 gram.)

PRINCIPLES OF CHEMISTRY UNDERLYING THE NURSING CARE

D. Definite amounts of water are essential to maintain the fluid balance of the body.

1. A true solution is a liquid mixture of ions, atoms, or molecules of 2 or more substances wherein there is apparent homogeneity.
   A. Water is by far the commonest and most useful solvent.
   B. The amounts of constituents in a solution may vary within certain limits.
2. Diffusion is a process wherein, because of molecular motion, 2 or more substances (gases, liquids, or solids) become perfectly mixed.
3. Osmosis is the process whereby the molecules of a solvent pass through a semi-permeable membrane from the area of lesser to greater concentration of the solute.
   A. A semi-permeable membrane is one which shows selective action with regard to the passage of different substances through it.
   B. Solvent molecules will pass through the semi-permeable membrane, because of osmosis, until the pressure exerted on the side of the formerly stronger solution is great enough to establish a state of equilibrium. The amount of pressure necessary to prevent the flow of solvent molecules across the membrane is called the osmotic pressure of the solution. (The greater the difference between the concentrations of the solutions on either side of the membrane, the greater the osmotic pressure will be.)
   C. An isotonic solution is one which exerts the same osmotic pressure as a solution on the other side of a semi-permeable membrane.
      (1) A hypotonic solution has less osmotic pressure, so

the solvent will pass through the membrane to the more concentrated solution on the opposite side.

(2) A hypertonic solution has a higher osmotic pressure so the solvent of the less concentrated solution will pass through the membrane to the hypertonic side.

(3) Physiological saline solution (isotonic with body fluids) is approximately a 0.9 per cent aqueous solution of sodium chloride.

4. Dialysis is the process wherein simple molecules or ions pass through a permeable membrane. (The size of the molecules allowed to pass through depends upon the permeability of the membrane.)

Section E: Nursing Care and Science Principles Related to Electrolyte Balance.

E. All the cells of the body require definite amounts of certain electrolytes for efficient functioning.

NURSING CARE

1. All patients should be observed for signs and symptoms of electrolyte imbalance, and these should be reported promptly. This is of particular importance when there is:
   A. Unusual loss of any body fluids which may be caused by:
      (1) Severe and/or prolonged vomiting or diarrhea.
      (2) Profuse perspiration.
      (3) Extensive burns.
      (4) Prolonged suction of gastric contents.
      (5) Some types of fistulae.
   B. A condition involving:
      (1) The adrenal cortex.
      (2) The pituitary gland.
      (3) The parathyroid glands (e.g. tumor or thyroidectomy).
      (4) Inadequate kidney function.
      (5) Inadequate nutrition.
   C. Administration of unusual amounts of fluids and/or electrolytes (especially when the urine flow is inadequate).
2. Reportable signs and symptoms of electrolyte imbalance may include:
   A. Signs and symptoms of edema or dehydration. (See Nursing Care Related to "D.")
   B. Abnormal breathing patterns (e.g. Kussmaul).

C. Signs and symptoms of hypotension. (See Nursing Care Related to "A.")
D. Muscular weakness, paralysis (including smooth muscle).
E. Muscular twitchings, tetany, cramping.
F. Fatigue, lethargy.
G. Signs and symptoms of damage to the brain (e.g. loss of consciousness).
H. Gastro-intestinal disturbances (e.g. nausea or anorexia).

3. When a patient has a condition in which electrolyte imbalance is a probability (e.g. Addison's disease),
   A. Orders should be sought concerning:
      (1) Dietary intake of electrolytes involved.
      (2) Fluid intake and output.
   B. Care should be taken to follow specifically medical orders pertaining to:
      (1) Dietary and fluid intake.
      (2) Saving of fluid output.
      (3) Weighing of patient.
   C. All fluid intake and output should be measured and reported.
4. Unless otherwise indicated, sodium intake may be encouraged when there is:
   A. Profuse perspiration.
   B. Loss of tissue fluid.
5. Measures to prevent severe and/or prolonged vomiting should be taken. (See Nursing Care Related to "C.")
6. Measures to prevent severe and/or prolonged diarrhea should be taken. (See Nursing Care Related to "C.")
7. Oral intake of fluids may be restricted when gastric contents are continually being removed by suction.
8. Only isotonic solutions of sodium chloride should be used for parenteral therapy unless the medical orders specify another concentration.
9. Extra calcium should be encouraged in the diets of growing children and pregnant women.

PRINCIPLES OF ANATOMY AND PHYSIOLOGY UNDERLYING THE NURSING CARE

E. All the cells of the body require definite amounts of certain electrolytes for efficient functioning.

1. Electrolytes are distributed in solution throughout all of the body fluids and cells.
   A. The primary cations are sodium, potassium, calcium and magnesium.
      (1) The chief cation in plasma is sodium.
      (2) The chief intracellular cation is potassium.
   B. The primary anions are chloride, bicarbonate, dihydrogen phosphate, sulfate and protein.
      (1) The chief anions in the plasma are chloride and bicarbonate.
      (2) The chief intracellular anions are bicarbonate and protein.
2. Electrolytes of body fluids:
   A. Contribute to proper osmotic pressure relationships.
   B. Provide buffer systems and mechanisms for regulating the acid-base balance.
   C. Provide proper ionic balance for normal tissue irritability and functioning.
   D. Often act as enzyme activators.
3. A major means for maintaining a constant concentration of electrolytes is the retention or elimination of water.
4. The total concentration of electrolytes in the body fluids is affected by total store of blood bicarbonate.
5. The kidney is an important organ in the regulation of electrolytic concentrations.
6. The reabsorption of sodium, potassium and chlorides in the kidney tubules is influenced by:
   A. Adrenal cortical hormone, which is responsible for the normal reabsorption of sodium and excretion of potassium. (Hyposecretion results in sodium loss and potassium retention.)
   B. Posterior pituitary (anti-diuretic hormone) which affects reabsorption through the reabsorption of water.

7. The body cells and fluids normally maintain an osmotic pressure of about 0.9 per cent sodium chloride. (Either hypotonic or hypertonic solutions in contact with cells may cause injury to the cells.)
8. Fixed anions are lost from the body primarily through the urine.
   A. Chloride ions may also be lost through loss of the gastric juices.
   B. Bicarbonate ions may also be lost through prolonged diarrhea.
9. Cations are lost primarily through the urine. (Sodium may also be lost in fairly large amounts through sweat, prolonged diarrhea or prolonged loss of gastric juices.)
10. Any excessive loss of body fluids may result in electrolyte imbalance.
11. A proper intracellular concentration of potassium is essential to normal cellular functioning.
    A. Potassium may be lost from the cells if:
       (1) Cell membranes are injured (e.g. in anoxia).
       (2) Acidosis exists.
       (3) There is an upset in sodium balance.
    B. Potassium deficiency may cause:
       (1) Lethargy.
       (2) Muscular weakness or paralysis.
       (3) Intestinal distention.
       (4) Changes in cardiac action.
12. A proper extracellular concentration of sodium is essential to:
    A. Fluid balance.
    B. Acid-base balance.
13. An adult needs a daily intake of 200 milligrams of sodium chloride to replace that normally lost through urine and perspiration.
14. Calcium is important in blood coagulation, bone formation, cardiac rhythmicity, maintenance of normal neuromuscular irritability and membrane permeability.
    A. A low serum calcium results in muscular twitchings, followed by jerking muscular contractions.

B. There is an increased need for calcium during growth, pregnancy and lactation.

C. Large amounts of calcium may be lost from the body in rickets, hypoparathyroidism and prolonged physical inactivity.

PRINCIPLES OF CHEMISTRY UNDERLYING THE NURSING CARE

E. All the cells of the body require definite amounts of certain electrolytes for efficient functioning.

1. An ion is a charged atom or group of atoms (caused by gain or loss of electrons).
   A. Strongly electro-positive elements form positive ions (e.g. potassium, sodium, calcium, magnesium).
   B. Strongly electro-negative elements form negative ions (e.g. fluorine, oxygen, chlorine).
2. Electrolytes are electrovalent compounds which, when in solution, form ions and will conduct electricity.
   A. Positively-charged ions are attracted to the negative pole, or cathode, and are called cations.
   B. Negatively-charged ions are attracted to the positive pole, or anode, and are called anions.
3. Osmosis is the process whereby the molecules of a solvent pass through a semi-permeable membrane from the area of lesser to greater concentration of the solute.
   A. A semi-permeable membrane is one which shows selective action with regard to the passage of different substances through it.
   B. Solvent molecules will pass through the semi-permeable membrane, because of osmosis, until the pressure exerted on the side of the formerly stronger solution is great enough to establish a state of equilibrium. The amount of pressure necessary to prevent the flow of solvent molecules across the membrane is called the osmotic pressure of the solution. (The greater the difference between the concentrations of the solutions of either side of the membrane, the greater the osmotic pressure will be.)

C. An isotonic solution is one which exerts the same osmotic pressure as a solution on the other side of a semi-permeable membrane.

(1) A hypotonic solution has less osmotic pressure, so the solvent will pass through the membrane to the more concentrated solution on the opposite side.

(2) A hypertonic solution has a higher osmotic pressure, so the solvent of the more dilute solution will pass through the membrane to the hypertonic side.

(3) Physiological saline solution (isotonic with body fluids) is approximately a 0.9 per cent aqueous solution of sodium chloride.

Section F: Nursing Care and Science Principles Related to the pH Environment.

F. All the cells of the body require a definite pH environment.

NURSING CARE

1. All patients should be observed for signs and symptoms of acid-base imbalance and these should be reported promptly. This is of particular importance when there is:
   A. Impaired circulation or respirations.
   B. Dehydration due to any cause.
   C. Severe and/or prolonged vomiting or diarrhea.
   D. Uncontrolled diabetes mellitus.
   E. Severe kidney damage.
   F. Administration of alkali or acids.
2. Reportable signs and symptoms of acid-base imbalance may include:
   A. Signs and symptoms of electrolyte imbalance. (See Nursing Care Related to "E.")
   B. Acetone odor on breath and ketonuria (when there is an accumulation of ketone bodies in the blood).
3. When a patient has a condition in which there is acid-base imbalance (e.g. diabetic coma),
   A. This should be handled as a medical emergency.
   B. Extreme care should be taken to follow specifically all orders involving:
      (1) The dietary or fluid intake.
      (2) The saving of fluid output.
   C. All fluid intake and output should be measured and reported.

D. Provision should be made for frequent testing of urine (e.g. equipment for acetone test, diacetic acid test on pH indicators).

E. Equipment should be made available for the intravenous administration of physiological saline solution, sodium bicarbonate solution, sodium lactate solution (or others as ordered).

4. When a patient has diabetes mellitus and acidosis occurs, equipment should be made available for the administration of large doses of crystalline insulin.
5. Emotional hyperventilation should be discouraged.

PRINCIPLES OF ANATOMY AND PHYSIOLOGY UNDERLYING THE NURSING CARE

F. All the cells of the body require a definite pH environment.

1. The value of the pH environment necessary for normal cellular functioning is about 7.4.
   A. Variations of even a few tenths may be fatal.
   B. To maintain this nearly neutral pH the basic and acid elements of the body must balance.
2. The proper pH of body fluids is maintained by the:
   A. Buffering action of various buffer systems such as those composed of:
      (1) Phosphate.
      (2) Bicarbonate.
      (3) Protein.
   B. Elimination of carbon dioxide in the lungs.
   C. Excretion of electrolytes by the kidneys.
3. The proper distribution of chloride and bicarbonate ions provides the primary means for maintaining the acid-base balance.
4. Practically all estimations of body acid-base balance are based upon the analysis of the bicarbonate buffer system. (The normal carbon dioxide combining power of plasma is 50 to 55 volumes per cent or 25 $\pm$ milli-equivalents.)
5. A fall in the pH of the blood may occur when there is:

A. An abnormal loss of bicarbonate ions from the body (e.g. in dehydration, diarrhea).
B. A relatively large and prolonged increase in acid metabolites (e.g. in diabetic coma or uremia).
   (1) Increased metabolism of fatty acids results in the excessive accumulation of ketone bodies in the blood (i.e. acetone, aceto-acetic acid and beta-hydroxybutyric acid).
   (2) Adequate carbohydrate metabolism prevents ketogenesis.
C. Toxicity due to drugs.

6. When there is a fall in the pH of the blood,
   A. The changed ratio of carbon dioxide concentration in the blood causes heavy forced breathing.
   B. The increased excretion of sodium causes diuresis.
   C. The pH change interferes with normal cellular functioning (e.g. brain damage with loss of consciousness).
   D. The resultant potassium imbalance results in problems of potassium deficiency.
   E. The urine becomes more acid (pH less than 5) because the kidneys excrete more chloride ions.
   F. Excessive amounts of ketone bodies produced by increased metabolism of fatty acids may be excreted in the urine. (Acetone may be excreted by the lungs, also.)
7. Acidosis may be lessened by:
   A. The administration of fluids.
   B. The administration of electrolytes, including sodium ions, potassium ions and/or bicarbonate ions.
   C. Treating the cause of the acidosis (e.g. insulin for diabetic).
8. A rise in the pH of the blood may occur when there is:
   A. Loss of chloride ions from the body (e.g. in severe and prolonged vomiting).
   B. Increased concentration of bicarbonate ions in the blood (e.g. in alkali therapy).
   C. Decreased concentration of carbon dioxide in the blood, such as may occur in hyperventilation.

9. When there is a rise in the pH of the blood,
   A. The changed ratio of carbon dioxide concentration in the blood causes slow, shallow respirations or periodic breathing patterns.
   B. The increased excretion of sodium causes diuresis.
   C. The urine becomes alkaline (pH more than 7.4) because the kidneys excrete more bicarbonate ions.
   D. The pH change interferes with normal cellular functioning (e.g. brain damage with loss of consciousness).
10. Alkalosis may be treated by:
   A. The administration of fluids.
   B. The administration of sodium and chloride ions.

PRINCIPLES OF CHEMISTRY UNDERLYING THE NURSING CARE

F. All the cells of the body require a definite pH environment.

1. Osmosis is the process whereby the molecules of a solvent pass through a semipermeable membrane from the area of lesser to greater concentration of the solute.
2. An ion is a charged atom or group of atoms (caused by gain or loss of electrons).
   A. Strongly electro-positive elements form positive ions (e.g. potassium, sodium, calcium or magnesium).
   B. Strongly electro-negative elements form negative ions (e.g. fluorine, oxygen, chlorine).
3. An acid may be defined as a compound which gives hydrogen ions (or hydronium ions) in solution.
4. A base may be defined as a compound which yields hydroxyl ions in solution.
5. The degree to which ionization to hydronium or hydroxyl ions occurs may be said to determine the strength of the acid or base. (Carbon dioxide dissolved in water forms carbonic acid which is a weak acid.)
6. The pH of a solution indicates the concentration of hydrogen ions present. It is stated as the negative of the logarithm of the hydrogen-ion concentration.
   A. Values above 7 indicate an increasingly basic solution.

B. Values below 7 indicate an increasingly acidic solution.
C. A pH of 7 indicates neutrality.

7. A pH indicator is a compound which has both acidic and basic forms, the colors of which are different, so that at particular pH values (specific for each indicator), there is a color change of the indicator. (Examples of pH indicators include litmus, phenolphthalein and nitrazene.)
8. A buffer system is a solution of a weak acid or base together with its salt which will retain its pH value upon the addition of small amounts of acid or base. (Examples of buffer systems include carbonic acid and sodium bicarbonate, phosphoric acid, and sodium acid phosphate.)
9. Acetone, a ketone, is a volatile liquid with a typical fruity odor.

Section G: Nursing Care and Science Principles Related to Enzymes and Hormones.

G. Normal body functioning is dependent upon the presence of certain enzymes and hormones.

NURSING CARE

1. All patients should be observed for signs and symptoms of hormonal imbalance and these should be reported. This is of particular importance when patients have problems involving:
   A. The thyroid gland.
   B. The parathyroid glands.
   C. The cortex of the adrenal gland.
   D. The islet cells of the pancreas.
   E. The pituitary gland.
2. Reportable signs and symptoms of hypothyroidism may include,
   A. In the child:
      (1) General lethargy, dullness.
      (2) Retardation of mental and physical growth.
      (3) Protruding tongue.
   B. In the adult:
      (1) General lethargy, dullness.
      (2) Dry, puffy skin.
      (3) Susceptibility to cold.
      (4) Amenorrhea or other menstrual irregularities.
      (5) Low pulse pressure.
      (6) Enlargement of thyroid gland.
3. When a patient has hypothyroidism, additional warmth should be provided as necessary.

4. Reportable signs and symptoms of hyperthyroidism may include:
   A. Nervousness, irritability, symptoms of anxiety (possibly symptoms of frank psychosis).
   B. Tremor, muscular weakness.
   C. Tachycardia.
   D. Dyspnea upon exertion.
   E. Hot, moist skin, increased sensitivity to heat.
   F. Excessive appetite accompanied by loss of weight.
   G. Exophthalmia.
   H. Enlargement of thyroid gland.
5. When a patient has hyperthyroidism,
   A. Provision should be made for adequate rest and sleep. (See Nursing Care Related to "J.")
   B. Physical exertion should be limited.
   C. Provision should be made for a comfortably cool external environment.
   D. Provision should be made for adequate nutritional intake (e.g. extra between-meal feedings).
   E. Provision should be made for emotional rest.
   F. Careful observations should be made for signs and symptoms of thyroid crisis and these should be reported immediately. These include:
      (1) A markedly elevated temperature.
      (2) Tachycardia.
      (3) Delirium, hyperactivity.
6. Reportable signs of hypoparathyroidism may include neuromuscular hyperexcitability with muscular twitchings and tetany.
7. When a patient has hypoparathyroidism,
   A. External stimuli should be limited.
   B. Equipment should be ready for the prompt intravenous administration of calcium if tetany occurs.
8. Reportable signs and symptoms of hyperparathyroidism may include:
   A. Fractures.
   B. Signs and symptoms of renal calculi (e.g. pain in kidney region or down into pelvis, hematuria).

9. When a patient has hyperparathyroidism,
   A. Care should be taken to prevent fractures. (See Nursing Care Related to "K.")
   B. Fluids should be encouraged within medical orders.
10. Reportable signs and symptoms of adrenal cortical insufficiency may include:
   A. Signs and symptoms of low blood pressure. (See Nursing Care Related to "A.")
   B. Abnormal pigmentation of the skin (bronzing).
   C. Poor response to cold.
   D. Signs and symptoms of electrolyte imbalance. (See Nursing Care Related to "E.")
11. Reportable signs and symptoms of too much adrenal cortical hormone may include:
   A. Moonface.
   B. High color or skin.
   C. Hirsutism in the female.
   D. Signs and symptoms of elevated blood pressure. (See Nursing Care Related to "A.")
   E. Mental aberrations.
12. When a patient has diabetes mellitus,
   A. He should be observed closely for signs and symptoms of hypo- and hyper-insulinism (the latter if he is on insulin therapy).
   B. Care should be taken to follow specifically all orders pertaining to diet, insulin and urine tests.
   C. Equipment should be available for the testing of urine for glucose, acetone and/or diacetic acid.
   D. All observations and test results should be reported.
13. Reportable signs and symptoms of hypoinsulinism may include:
   A. The diabetic triad of:
      (1) Polydypsia.
      (2) Polyuria.
      (3) Polyphagia.
   B. Weakness.
   C. Glycosuria (possibly accompanied by pruritis).

D. Signs and symptoms of acidosis. (See Nursing Care Related to "F.")

14. Reportable signs and symptoms of hyperinsulinism may include:
    A. Hunger.
    B. Weakness, drowsiness.
    C. Hyper-excitability, nervousness, headache.
    D. Dizziness.
    E. Pallor.
    F. Profuse perspiration.
    G. Convulsions.
    H. Loss of consciousness.
15. When there is a possibility of hyperinsulinism occurring,
    A. Orders should be sought concerning any immediate treatment.
    B. Glucose in a form which can be absorbed rapidly should be readily available (e.g. corn syrup, sugar candies, or orange juice).
    C. The patient should be closely observed during hours in which this condition is most likely to occur (depends greatly upon the type of insulin administered).
16. When symptoms of hyperinsulinism occur, a glucose preparation should be administered immediately (e.g. a glass of orange juice, a small amount of corn syrup).
    A. If this treatment fails to remedy the condition, the doctor should be notified promptly.
    B. If mealtime is more than an hour away and/or the patient has had a slow acting insulin, an order may be sought to give a carbohydrate food which will be absorbed slowly (e.g. milk).
17. Obesity should be reported.
18. Lack of development of secondary sex characteristics should be reported.
19. When pitocin is administred to a pregnant woman at term, she should be observed closely for severe, prolonged uterine contractions. If this occurs:
    A. It should be reported promptly.

B. The pitocin should be discontinued until ordered further.
C. A general anesthetic should be prepared for use as ordered.

PRINCIPLES OF ANATOMY AND PHYSIOLOGY UNDERLYING THE NURSING CARE

G. Normal body functioning is dependent upon the presence of certain enzymes and hormones.

Facts Related to Enzymes

1. An enzyme is an organic catalyst produced by a living organism.
2. Enzymes play important roles in such body processes as:
   A. The digestion and absorption of food.
   B. The metabolism of carbohydrates, fats and proteins.
   C. Intracellular oxidations and reductions.
   D. Muscle contractions.
   E. Blood clotting.

Facts Related to Hormones

1. Hormones are secreted by specific glandular cells and are carried by the blood or lymph to organs or tissues where they influence various body functions.
2. The thyroid hormone helps to regulate the metabolic rate, primarily through affecting cellular oxidation.
   A. The active principle, thyroxin, contains a high percentage of iodine.
   B. Hyposecretion of thyroxin in childhood may result in:
      (1) Mental and physical retardation.
      (2) Retarded reproductive activities.
      (3) Generalized hypofunctioning of cells (low metabolic rate).
   C. Hyposecretion in the adult may result in:
      (1) Apathy, lethargy.
      (2) Generalized edema of subcutaneous tissues.
      (3) Susceptibility to cold.
      (4) Changes in reproductive functions (e.g. menstrual irregularities).

(5) Generalized hypofunctioning of cells (low metabolic rate).
(6) Adiposity.

D. Hypersecretion (or overdosage) results in an increased metabolic rate which may be accompanied by:
(1) Nervousness.
(2) Muscular weakness, tremors.
(3) Tachycardia.
(4) Hot, moist skin and increased sensitivity to heat.
(5) Loss of weight.
(6) Exophthalmia.
(7) Dyspnea upon exertion (due to oxygen deficiency).

E. Extreme symptoms of hypersecretion occur in a thyroid crisis.

F. Hyperplasia of the thyroid gland may occur in hypothyroidism or hyperthyroidism.

G. There is a reciprocal relationship between the amount of thyrotropic hormone produced in the anterior pituitary and the amount of hormone produced by the thyroid gland.

3. The parathyroid hormone affects calcium and phosphorus metabolism.
   A. Hyposecretion may result in hypocalcemia which causes neuromuscular hyper-excitability. (Severe tetany can result in death from asphyxiation.)
   B. The parathyroid glands lie close to or are embedded in the thyroid gland.
   C. Hypersecretion (or overdosage) may result in:
   (1) Decalcification of bone.
   (2) Hypercalcemia which may cause renal calculi.
4. The adrenal medulla secretes adrenalin which causes:
   A. An increase in the stroke volume of the heart.
   B. Some peripheral vaso-constriction.
   C. Bronchiolar dilatation.
   D. Increased glycogenolysis.
5. Impulses from the hypothalamus can cause the discharge of adrenalin into the blood stream (e.g. emotional response to fear or excitement).

6. The adrenal cortex secretes hormones which are concerned with:
   A. The metabolism of sodium, potassium, chlorides and water (essential to life).
   B. The metabolism of carbohydrates and protein.
   C. Adaptation to stress.
   D. Sexual development (to limited extent).
7. Hyposecretion of these hormones may result in:
   A. Hypotension.
   B. Muscular weakness.
   C. Poor response to cold or other stress situations.
   D. Gastro-intestinal disturbances (e.g. anorexia, vomiting).
   E. Abnormal pigmentation of the skin.
   F. Feminism in the male.
8. Hypersecretion (or overdosage) of these hormones may result in:
   A. Hypertension.
   B. Mental aberrations.
   C. Symptoms of metabolic disturbance (e.g. obesity or edema).
   D. Virilism in the female.
9. There is a reciprocal relationship between the amount of ACTH produced in the anterior pituitary and the amount of cortical hormones produced in the adrenal gland.
10. The islet cells of the pancreas secrete insulin.
    A. Insulin is involved in the metabolism of glucose and is essential to:
       (1) The normal storage of glycogen.
       (2) The oxidation of glucose.
    B. The normal glucose level in the blood is 70 to 100 mgm. per cent. (Brain cells can metabolize only glucose for energy.)
    C. Hypersecretion (or overdosage) may result in hypoglycemia with the following symptoms:
       (1) Hunger, mild nausea, weakness, drowsiness, hyperexcitability, nervousness, headache, pallor and profuse perspiration (early symptoms).

(2) Mild to severe convulsions, confusion (late symptoms).
(3) Coma and death.

D. Hyposecretion of insulin (or inactivation of insulin or insufficient dosage) may result in
(1) Decreased metabolism of glucose with hyperglycemia which cause the following:
(a) Glycosuria accompanied by polyuria.
(b) Thirst.
(c) Hunger.
(d) Weakness.
(2) Increased metabolism of fatty acids with the production of ketone bodies which give rise to:
(a) Acidosis.
(b) Ketonuria.
(c) Acetone breath.
(3) Increased metabolism of proteins with wasting of the body, if prolonged.
(4) Peripheral arterial disease with deposits of cholesterol in the arteries, if prolonged.

11. The ovaries produce estrogens and progesterone which are necessary for the development of secondary sex characteristics and normal reproductive functions in the female.
12. There are reciprocal relationships between the amounts of follicle-stimulating hormone and interstitial cell-stimulating hormone produced in the anterior pituitary and the amount of ovarian hormones produced.
13. The testes produce androgens (active principle, testosterone) which are necessary for the development of secondary sex characteristics and normal reproductive functions in the male.
14. Follicle-stimulating hormone produced in the anterior pituitary influences the maturation of spermatozoa and the interstitial cell stimulating hormone influences the production of testosterone.
15. The anterior pituitary gland produces somatotropins which affect growth and metabolic functions.

A. Hyposecretion may result in dwarfism or other metabolic disturbances (e.g. Simmonds' disease).

B. Hypersecretion may result in:
   (1) Gigantism in childhood.
   (2) Acromegaly in adulthood.
   (3) Other metabolic disturbances (e.g. Cushing's syndrome).

16. The posterior pituitary gland produces:
   A. An anti-diuretic factor.
   B. Pressor substances, including:
      (1) Vaso-pressor substance.
      (2) An oxytocic principle which causes smooth muscle contraction in the gastro-intestinal tract and the gravid uterus at term.

PRINCIPLES OF CHEMISTRY UNDERLYING THE NURSING CARE

G. Normal body functioning is dependent upon the presence of certain enzymes and hormones.

1. A catalyst is a substance which speeds a chemical reaction but does not change permanently itself in the reaction.
2. Oxidation-reduction reactions involve the transference of electrons. Atoms which gain electrons are reduced and atoms which lose electrons are oxidized. (The oxidation of carbon and hydrogen in foodstuffs by oxygen is an energy-liberating chemical reaction and when oxidation is complete, carbon dioxide and water are produced.)
3. The amount of solute which can be dissolved in a given amount of liquid may vary within certain limits. (After the saturation point has been reached, additional solute cannot be dissolved.)
4. Starch is a polysaccharide which can be hydrolyzed to the disaccharide, maltose.
5. Maltose, sucrose, and lactose are disaccharides which can be hydrolyzed to monosaccharides.
   A. Maltose can be hydrolyzed to glucose.
   B. Sucrose can be hydrolyzed to glucose and fructose.
   C. Lactose can be hydrolyzed to glucose and galactose.
6. Acetone, a ketone, is a volatile liquid with a typical fruity odor.

Section H: Nursing Care and Science Principles Related to the Body Temperature.

H. There is a definite temperature range for efficient cellular functioning and proper enzymatic activity.

NURSING CARE

1. Patients should be observed for signs and symptoms of abnormal body temperature and these should be reported. This is of particular importance when the patient:
   A. Has an infection.
   B. Has brain injury (especially when there is loss of consciousness).
   C. Has any major body injury (e.g. surgery).
   D. Has severe skin destruction.
   E. Has thyrotoxicosis.
   F. Has a deficiency in mature white blood cells.
   G. Has impaired general circulation.
   H. Is a premature or sick infant or a young child.
   I. Is receiving a blood transfusion or other intravenous therapy.
   J. Is exposed to extremes of external temperatures.
   K. Is having fever therapy.
   L. Is having chills.
2. Reportable signs and symptoms of an elevated body temperature may include:
   A. An oral temperature above 99° F. (Rectal 100° F.) (An oral or rectal temperature of 104° F. or above should always be reported promptly.)
   B. A rapid full pulse to rapid weak pulse.

C. Hyperemia of skin (may be preceded by a pale skin).
D. Profuse sweating.
E. Hot, dry skin.
F. Rapid respirations (may be panting).
G. Feeling of warmth (may be preceded by chills).
H. Headache, general malaise, restlessness and irritability, mental confusion, loss of consciousness.
I. Convulsions (seen frequently in children).

3. Signs and symptoms of a lowered body temperature may include:
   A. An oral temperature below 95° F. (Rectal 96° F.)
   B. Rapid full pulse to slow, weak pulse.
   C. Paleness or cyanosis of skin.
   D. Slow respirations.
   E. "Goosebumps" on skin.
   F. Shivering, chattering of teeth.
   G. Feeling of coldness.
   H. Excessive coldness, pain, followed by numbness and loss of sensation.
4. Rectal temperature should be taken in preference to oral temperature when:
   A. The patient is not responsible.
   B. A most nearly accurate measurement of body temperature is important (e.g. in generalized infections or in brain injuries).
   C. The patient has a tube through his mouth or nose.
   D. The patient has had oral or nasal surgery.
   E. The patient has a dental plate in place and an accurate measurement is desired.
5. Oral or axillary temperatures should be taken in preference to rectal measurements when the patient:
   A. Has had rectal, perineal or anal surgery.
   B. Has diarrhea or constipation.
6. Oral temperatures should not be taken within 30 minutes after the patient has eaten or drunk hot or cold food or fluids.
7. Body temperature should be evaluated in relation to such factors as:

A. The usual body temperature.
B. The time of day.
C. The environmental temperature.
D. The amount of physical activity.
E. The phase of the menstrual cycle.
F. The course of illness.

8. Particular attention should be paid to the control of the external temperature and/or supplying or avoiding external warmth when the patient has:
   A. Impaired peripheral circulation.
   B. Skin destruction (e.g. burns).
   C. Thyroid disturbance.
   D. Abnormal body weight.
   E. Decreased sensory perception of temperature.
   F. General physical fatigue.
   G. Limited muscular activity.
   H. Age extremes (premature infant and very aged).
9. When a patient has an elevated temperature (not artificially induced),
   A. The external environmental temperature should be adjusted to be cooler.
   B. Muscular activity should be limited.
   C. Fluids should be encouraged (within medical orders).
   D. Loss of body heat by radiation, conduction, or evaporation may be encouraged (e.g. water or alcohol sponges as ordered and/or indicated, removal of blankets or use of fan).
   E. Easily digested meals should be given.
   F. External friction should be avoided.
   G. Anti-pyretic drugs may be administered as ordered for this symptom.
   H. The body temperature should be checked frequently (e.g. every 15 minutes to every 4 hours).
   I. Chilling should be avoided (except in cases of extremely high temperature).
10. When a patient has a lowered temperature,
    A. The external environmental temperature should be adjusted to be warmer.

B. Muscular activity may be encouraged (in accord with condition).
C. Warm foods and fluids may be encouraged.
D. Loss of body heat by radiation, conduction or evaporation should be discouraged (e.g. use of blankets or protection from draughts).
E. External warmth may be added with use of applications of heat as ordered.
F. The body temperature should be checked frequently (e.g. from every hour to every 4 hours).

PRINCIPLES OF ANATOMY AND PHYSIOLOGY UNDERLYING THE NURSING CARE

H. There is a definite temperature range for efficient cellular functioning and proper enzymatic activity.

1. Body cells vary in their abilities to function when the temperature is below 95° F. (Normal functioning of the cells of the central nervous system is impossible at a temperature above 106° F.)
2. The optimum temperature for normal activity of enzymes falls within the normal body temperature range.
3. The normal range of oral temperature is 96° F. to 99° F.
   A. Rectal temperatures may be close to 1° higher. (A body temperature measured rectally will not be accurate unless the thermometer is in contact with mucosal lining of the rectum.)
   B. Axillary temperatures may be close to 1° lower.
   C. There is a diurnal variation of temperature. (If the waking hours are during the day, the maximum temperature is in the late afternoon and the minimum in the early morning.)
   D. There may be a rise in temperature (0.3° to 1° F.) from the time of ovulation until menstruation (or through pregnancy).
   E. The temperatures of infants and young children fluctuate easily.
   F. Oral temperatures may be influenced by:

(1) The previous oral intake of hot or cold food or fluids.
(2) Mouth breathing.

4. The body temperature represents a balance between heat produced in the tissues (and that acquired from the external environment) and heat lost to the environment.
5. Heat production is due to exothermic chemical reactions which are increased by such factors as:
   A. Generalized increased metabolic rate (e.g. when there is hyperthyroidism).
   B. Muscular exercise.
   C. A cold environmental temperature.
6. The amount of heat lost from the body surface by radiation and conduction varies with:
   A. The amount of body insulation (e.g. subcutaneous fat, clothing).
   B. The amount of skin area exposed.
   C. The external environmental temperature.
   D. The amount of blood flow in the peripheral capillaries.
7. The amount of heat lost from the body surface by vaporization depends upon:
   A. The production of sweat.
   B. The amount of skin area exposed.
   C. The amount of blood flow in the peripheral capillaries.
   D. The humidity of the surrounding atmosphere.
   E. The air currents.
8. Body heat is distributed throughout the body by:
   A. Conduction through the tissues.
   B. The circulating blood.
9. The total amount of heat in a given area is influenced by the rate of blood flow.
   A. Peripheral vaso-constriction results in decreased heat loss (cold skin).
   B. Peripheral vasodilatation results in increased heat loss (warm skin).
10. When the body loses more heat than it can produce in the basal state, shivering and gooseflesh appear.

11. The physiological mechanisms for temperature regulation are controlled by nerve centers in the hypothalamus.
    A. Heat-regulating mechanisms are generally not fully developed at birth. (Variations of as much as 2 degrees may occur quite spontaneously during the first year of life.)
    B. Autonomic nerves regulate vaso-constriction, sweat gland activity and contraction of the arrector pili muscles.
12. Heat regulation mechanisms are depressed by some drugs (e.g. alcohol, morphine or general anesthetics), sleep and general fatigue.
13. Heat loss may be increased by increased diaphoresis (e.g. use of aspirin or after exercise).
14. Toxins of some infective agents and other chemicals (e.g. hemoglobin) in the body may act on the temperature-regulating centers (directly or indirectly) to raise the threshold for mechanisms operating to increase heat loss.
    A. The first reaction is a decrease in heat loss with peripheral vaso-constriction and a sensation of chilling which may be accompanied by shivering.
    B. The second reaction is increased heat production followed eventually by peripheral vaso-dilatation and an uncomfortably warm sensation.

PRINCIPLES OF PHYSICS UNDERLYING THE NURSING CARE

H. There is a definite temperature range for efficient cellular functioning and proper enzymatic activity.

1. Evaporation is the process whereby a substance in liquid state is changed to a vapor state and this process requires heat. (Evaporation is a cooling process.)
2. Heat can be defined as the kinetic energy of molecules.
    A. Heat travels from a point of higher temperature to one of lower temperature.
    B. Conduction is the transmission of heat through any substance.

C. Radiation is the transmission of heat through a vacuum (space).

D. Convection is the transmission of heat by the movement of a heated liquid or gas. (Because of convection, increasing air movements will increase the loss of heat from an object.)

3. Friction changes mechanical energy to thermal energy.

PRINCIPLES OF CHEMISTRY UNDERLYING THE NURSING CARE

H. There is a definite temperature range for efficient cellular functioning and proper enzymatic activity.

1. Exothermic chemical reactions are those in which there is a liberation of heat.

Section I: Nursing Care and Science Principles Related to Elimination.

I. Efficient body functioning requires that the food residues and gases in the gastro-intestinal tract be eliminated and that toxic substances formed in the body be rendered harmless and/or be eliminated.

NURSING CARE

1. All patients should be observed for anuria and oliguria and these should be reported. This is of particular importance when there is:
   A. Kidney disease.
   B. A problem of fluid imbalance.
2. When oliguria, anuria or high blood urea nitrogen occur, the patient should be observed closely for signs and symptoms of electrolyte imbalance. (See Nursing Care Related to "E.")
3. The urine should be observed for color, tranparency, sediment and odor and abnormalities should be reported.
4. All patients should be observed for signs and symptoms of jaundice and these should be reported. This is of particular importance when there is question of liver disease. (Reportable signs and symptoms of jaundice include:
   A. Yellow tinge of sclera and skin.
   B. Itching.
   C. Dark brown urine.
   D. Clay-colored stools.
5. All patients should be observed for signs and symptoms of

decreased bowel elimination and these should be reported. This is of particular importance when there is:

A. Paralysis or immobilization below the waist.
B. A disease condition or surgical condition involving the gastro-intestinal tract.
C. Dehydration.
D. Physical inactivity (e.g. prolonged bed rest).
E. Old age.
F. Pregnancy.
G. General depression of body functions such as may occur in mental depression, in myxedema or when narcotics are being taken.
H. Diagnostic examination of the gastro-intestinal tract requiring the use of barium.
I. Inability to communicate.

6. Observations of the amount and type of bowel elimination should be evaluated in relation to:
   A. The individual's usual pattern for bowel elimination.
   B. The amount and type of diet.
   C. The state of fluid balance.
7. Reportable signs and symptoms of decreased bowel elimination may include:
   A. Headache, general malaise, loss of appetite.
   B. Abdominal pain, cramping, feeling of pressure.
   C. Abdominal distention.
   D. Small amounts of hard stool.
   E. Stool retention with small amounts of liquid stool.
   F. Stools of narrow caliber.
8. Good bowel elimination may be aided by:
   A. Encouraging regularity of bowel habits.
   B. Providing for bowel evacuation when the urge to defecate exists.
   C. Providing for as close to usual posture for defecation as is possible.
   D. Encouraging fluids.
   E. Providing for physical activity.
   F. Encouraging a well-balanced diet with adequate roughage.

G. Providing for foods which tend to have a laxative effect on the individual.
H. Recognizing possible emotional components and giving supportive care accordingly.
I. Discouraging continued use of laxatives or enemas unless ordered by physician.
J. Reporting problems with bowel elimination.
K. Administering laxatives or enemas as ordered.

9. Flatulence may be decreased by:
   A. Encouraging the individual to expel gas voluntarily.
   B. Physical activity.
   C. Changes of position.
   D. Use of rectal tube (unless contraindicated).
   E. Use of enemas as ordered.
   F. Use of gastric or intestinal suction as ordered.
   G. Discouraging swallowing of air.
   H. Bubbling of baby during and after feedings.
   I. Encouraging the ingestion of solid foods (when permitted).
10. Incontinence of feces (after bowel control is learned) should be reported.

PRINCIPLES OF ANATOMY AND PHYSIOLOGY UNDERLYING THE NURSING CARE

I. Efficient body functioning requires that the food residues and gases in the gastro-intestinal tract be eliminated and that toxic substances formed in the body be rendered harmless and/or be eliminated.

1. The kidneys and lungs eliminate most of the waste products of cellular metabolism.
   A. Most of the nitrogenous wastes (result of protein metabolism) are eliminated in the urine.
      (1) The organic compounds include urea, uric acid and creatinine. (The liver plays the predominant role in the formation of urea.)
      (2) The most abundant inorganic compound is ammonia which is eliminated in ammonium salts.

(3) Kidney function normally keeps the blood urea nitrogen level below 20 mg. per cent.

B. To be excreted by the kidneys, solids must be in solution.

C. Carbon dioxide is eliminated through the lungs.

D. Pregnant women also excrete the waste products from the metabolic processes of the fetus.

2. Renal insufficiency may result in a general disturbance of the electrolyte and fluid balances. (The "uremic state" is generally preceded by anuria or oliguria, urine with low specific gravity and a rise in the blood urea nitrogen level.)
3. The skin, through the activity of the sweat glands, also excretes many compounds found in urine.
4. The liver excretes bile pigments. (Liver damage may be indicated by jaundice.)
5. The liver detoxifies many injurious substances (e.g. products of intestinal putrefaction and intermediate products of metabolism).
6. Much of the water of the intestinal contents is absorbed in the large intestine.
   A. If the body is dehydrated, absorption will be increased. (Some colons tend to absorb water very readily.)
   B. Retention of feces leads to increased absorption of water.
   C. Increased intestinal motility decreases the amount of water absorption.
7. The feces contain bacteria, sloughed-off epithelial cells, food residues, bile pigments, mucus and some inorganic salts.
   A. The volume of feces is increased by indigestible matter (e.g. cellulose).
   B. In starvation the bulk of the feces is reduced.
   C. Bile pigments give a brown color to the feces.
   D. The color varies to some extent with the food eaten.
8. The sudden passage of feces into the rectum initiates the defecatory reflex.
   A. The act of defecation can usually be inhibited by voluntarily constricting the external anal sphincter. (Exceptions occur when pressure due to intestinal peristalsis is greater than that produced by sphincter constriction, when the motor nerves which stimulate the sphincter are

undeveloped or injured or when the sphincter muscles are injured. The anal sphincter muscles can be torn during childbirth.)

B. The rectum may become tolerant to the presence of increased fecal bulk, and the desire to defecate may pass.

9. Atony of the muscular wall of the large intestine may occur:
   A. When fecal bulk is retained.
   B. In old age.
   C. When parasympathetic stimulation is decreased (e.g. when some drugs are administered or in some emotional states).
   D. When laxatives or enemas have been used for prolonged periods of time.
10. Spasms of the colon, causing obstruction in the passage of intestinal contents, may result from:
    A. Reflex irritation from injured abdominal viscera.
    B. Greatly increased parasympathetic stimulation (e.g. when some drugs are administered or in some emotional states).
    C. Irritation of the bowel (e.g. from laxatives).
11. The effect of different foodstuffs upon motility of the intestinal tract varies in individuals.
12. Bowel movements may occur, normally, as frequently as several times a day or as infrequently as once or twice a week.
13. External pressure exerted on the rectum and sigmoid by strong contraction of the diaphragm and abdominal muscles may help in the defecation process.
14. Ribbon-like stools or stools of narrow caliber may indicate lower intestinal obstruction.
15. Prolonged internal pressure against the walls of the rectum and sigmoid may cause headache and lethargy.
16. Sensory nerve endings for pain and pressure in the bowel wall may be stimulated by spasm of the smooth muscle of the bowel and by bowel distention.
17. Gas in the gastro-intestinal tract is primarily swallowed air. (Small amounts of other gases may be formed from intestinal putrefaction and/or fermentation.)

18. Gases may be eliminated from the gastro-intestinal tract by:
    A. Belching.
    B. Passing of flatus through the rectum.

PRINCIPLES OF CHEMISTRY UNDERLYING THE NURSING CARE

I. Efficient body functioning requires that the food residues and gases in the gastro-intestinal tract be eliminated and that toxic substances formed in the body be rendered harmless and/or be eliminated.

1. The chemical breakdown of hemoglobin involves the breakdown of heme to bilirubin (red) which can be oxidized to biliverdin (green) which can, in turn, be reduced to stercobilin (brown).
2. Barium sulfate, a salt relatively opaque to x-ray, is insoluble in water.
3. Fermentation is a chemical process in which carbohydrates are decomposed by the action of micro-organisms and bubbles of gas often develop as the organisms form carbon dioxide and hydrogen gases.
4. Putrefaction is a chemical process in which proteins are decomposed by the action of micro-organisms and several gaseous products often develop (e.g. hydrogen sulfide).

Section J: Nursing Care and Science Principles Related to Rest and Sleep.

J. Body cells require periods of decreased activity during which they can restore themselves.

NURSING CARE

1. All patients should be observed for the quality and quantity of their sleep and rest, and abnormal deviations should be reported.
2. Sleep and rest may be evaluated in relation to:
   A. The usual sleep pattern.
   B. Age.
   C. The general physical and emotional condition.
   D. Any drugs which have been administered.
3. Reportable signs and symptoms of insufficient sleep and rest may include:
   A. Loss of muscle tone, incoordination.
   B. Dizziness.
   C. Dark circles under the eyes and puffiness around the eyes.
   D. Reddened and burning conjunctiva, ptosis of eyelids.
   E. Yawning.
   F. Irritability.
   G. Lassitude.
   H. Inability to concentrate.
4. When an individual is in a stress-producing situation (e.g. illness, hospitalization or pregnancy), rest and sleep may be encouraged.
5. Sleep and rest may be encouraged by:
   A. Providing for a non-stimulating environment (e.g. limiting light or sound).
   B. Providing for physical comfort. (See Nursing Care Related to "N.")

C. Providing for psychological comfort.
D. Providing for muscular relaxation. (See Nursing Care Related to "K.")
E. Providing for both physical and mental activities and varieties of each during a 24-hour period.
F. Administration of sedative or hypnotic drugs as ordered.

PRINCIPLES OF ANATOMY AND PHYSIOLOGY UNDERLYING THE NURSING CARE

J. Body cells require periods of decreased activity during which they can restore themselves.

1. The required hours of sleep and rest vary with each individual.
   A. The average number of required hours of sleep include the following:
      (1) For infants, 18 to 20 hours.
      (2) For children, 10 to 14 hours.
      (3) For adults, 7 to 9 hours.
      (4) For elderly people, 5 to 7 hours.
   B. Sleep patterns are learned.
2. During sleep the metabolic rate is reduced below the basal level. (Deep sleep is more restful than light sleep.)
3. The higher the metabolic rate, the greater is the need for increased circulation, respirations, nutrition and excretion. (Muscular activity increases the metabolic rate.)
4. Decreasing the demands placed upon the body during a stress situation allows for greater total body response to the stress.
5. Energy is required both for responding to a stimulus and repressing response to a stimulus.
6. Factors which interfere with sleep and rest include:
   A. Discomfort.
   B. Impulses from visual, auditory or cutaneous receptors.
   C. Cortical activity (e.g. from psychic causes). (Anxiety is a frequent cause of sleeplessness.)
7. Inability to sleep may be accompanied by restlessness, hyperactivity and muscular tension.

Section K: Nursing Care and Science Principles Related to the Bones, Muscles and Joints.

K. The muscular and skeletal systems provide a means of locomotion, support for body structures and protection for soft tissues.

NURSING CARE

1. All patients should be observed for signs and symptoms of injury to the muscular and skeletal systems or to structures of the nervous system concerned with voluntary muscle activity, and these should be reported. This is of particular importance when a patient:
   A. Is a newborn.
   B. Has been in an accident (e.g. falling or automobile accident).
   C. Has a disease or surgical condition involving the bones, muscles or joints (e.g. arthritis).
   D. Has a disease condition or injury involving the brain, spinal cord, peripheral nerves or kinesthetic receptors.
   E. Has restricted physical activity (e.g. prolonged bedrest).
   F. Is pregnant or has borne children.
2. Reportable signs and symptoms of injury to the muscular and skeletal systems may include:
   A. Change in contour, alignment or contiguity of part or parts.
   B. Loss of or change in function of an affected part.
   C. Crepitus.
   D. Muscle spasm.
   E. Pain.
   F. Swelling.

G. Discoloration of skin (e.g. hematoma).
H. Difficulty in breathing (if thorax affected).

3. Reportable signs and symptoms of injury to the motor nerves, kinesthetic receptors or sensory nerves for pressure may include:
   A. A paralysis (flaccid or spastic).
   B. Convulsions, tics, spasms, tremors.
   C. Changes in muscular movements (e.g. in strength or co-ordination).
   D. Hypoactive reflexes (e.g. loss of knee jerk).
   E. Hyperactive reflexes (e.g. ankle clonus or tonic neck reflex).
4. All patients should be protected from mechanical injury to the muscular and skeletal systems and to the peripheral nerves.
   A. Patients should be provided and encouraged to maintain the closest approach possible to normal anatomical alignment while in any posture (lying, sitting, standing) and, when normal alignment is not possible, effort should be directed toward improving the alignment (e.g. through positioning, adjustment of equipment or environmental factors).
   B. Patients may be taught and should be encouraged to use principles of good body mechanics.
      (1) The body should be balanced over a firm base of support in standing, walking, squatting or rising. (Using a wide stance and keeping the body centered over the base of support increases stability of an upright posture.)
      (2) When carrying heavy objects the balance of the body should be shifted from the ankle rather than from the trunk.
      (3) Prolonged carrying of objects on one side should be avoided.
      (4) The pelvis and lower extremities should provide a firm support for the vertebral column (e.g. use of low-heeled shoes or standing and walking postures which provide this support).

(5) The least amount of muscular effort necessary to perform a given task should be used.
  (a) Movements should be made smoothly and rhythmically.
  (b) In lifting or carrying heavy objects, the arms should be held close to the body and the object should be close to the body before lifting is done.
  (c) When moving a heavy object, the parts of the body should be placed in such a way as to face in the same direction as the force to be applied.
  (d) Objects should be moved or slid along surfaces if possible, rather than lifted.
  (e) Body weight should be utilized whenever possible to push or pull objects.
  (f) When performing tasks, the sitting position should be used in preference to standing whenever possible.
  (g) Work levels should be such that muscle strain is minimized.

(6) Objects which are too heavy to be moved alone should not be lifted without adequate assistance.

(7) The muscles best suited to the task to be done should be utilized.
  (a) In lifting, pushing or pulling the muscles of the lower extremities should be used rather than the muscles of the trunk.
  (b) In carrying heavy objects, the muscles of the upper extremities should be used rather than the muscles of the trunk.
  (c) When reaching upward or working at low levels, the trunk should be maintained in normal alignment and adjustments made by the lower extremities (e.g. rising on toes or squatting).

C. Patients should be encouraged to use proper wearing apparel and this should be provided as necessary and/or possible.

(1) Clothing should not add heavy weight or pull over the shoulders.

(2) Brassieres should be well-fitting, providing uplift and firm support for the breasts.

(3) Foundation garments should be well-fitting and constructed for the purpose for which they are worn (e.g. corsets or braces).

(4) Shoes and hosiery should be of the correct length and width.

(5) High heels should be discouraged for regular wear (of great importance for pregnant women).

D. The major body joints should be moved (actively or passively) through their normal and/or anatomically possible ranges of motion *only* and this should be done at least once daily. (These include the freely movable joints of the trunk and extremities.)

(1) For complete abduction of the shoulder, the humerus must be outwardly rotated after the first 90 degrees of motion.

(2) Flexion of the fingers can best be accomplished when the wrist is in hyperextension and the flexion should allow for the natural deviation of the fingers toward the thumb side of the palm.

E. Patients should have normal or physiologically possible active exercise of the major groups of muscles daily unless this is contraindicated.

(1) These include the flexors and extensors of the toes and fingers; the flexors, extensors and rotators of the feet and hands, the extensors of the legs and thighs; the flexors, extensors, supinators and pronators of the lower arm; the flexors, extensors and rotators of the upper arm; the extensors of the vertebral column; the interscapular muscles and the abdominal musculature.

(2) Exercise should be increased gradually.

(3) Patients should be encouraged to assume activities of daily living as possible.

F. The body parts (e.g. shoulders, knees, elbows, feet and vertebral column) should be provided adequate support without pressure, drag or strain. This is of particular importance for:
 (1) Infants and young children.
 (2) The elderly.
 (3) Patients who are inactive for prolonged periods of time.
 (4) Patients who have lost consciousness or have loss of sensory perception for pressure.

G. An intramuscular injection should not exceed 2 to 3 cc. in the deltoid or 5 to 8 cc. in the gluteus maximum.
 (1) The size of the muscle and the type of drug injected should be considered, also, in determining the amount to administer in a single injection.
 (2) When the gluteus maximus muscle is used for an intramuscular injection, the injection should be made in the upper outer quadrant.

H. Patients should have frequent (e.g. at least 3 times daily) changes of position within medical orders.

I. Patients should be moved smoothly and the body parts should be maintained in alignment during the process.

J. The body and its parts should be handled firmly but gently.

K. All patients should be protected from accidents which could cause mechanical injury (e.g. with use of side rails, safe equipment, padding of beds or support of weakened muscles), and this is of particular importance when the patient:
 (1) Is not responsible.
 (2) Is subject to or is having convulsions.
 (3) Is subject to or has loss of consciousness.
 (4) Has difficulty with equilibrium (e.g. has injury to midbrain, cerebellum, vestibular apparatus, or has visual or auditory disturbance).
 (5) Has loss of kinesthetic sense.
 (6) Is blind.
 (7) Has limited motor ability.

(8) Has poor bone structure or strength.
(9) Has open fontanels.

L. Caution should be observed in the use of manual artificial respirations and this is of particular importance in infants, young children and elderly people.

M. Straining at stool should be discouraged. (See Nursing Care Related to "I.")

5. When injury to the skull has occurred (or is suspected),

A. The patient should be kept in horizontal position (unless ordered otherwise).

B. The head may be immobilized (e.g. with use of sandbags).

C. Any sudden, quick head movements should be prevented.

D. Pressure against the injured part should be prevented.

E. The patient should be observed closely for:

(1) Changes in blood pressure and rate and quality of pulse associated with increasing intracranial pressure.
(2) Signs and symptoms of shock. (See Nursing Care Related to "A.")
(3) Bleeding from the ears and nose.
(4) Leakage of cerebrospinal fluid.
(5) Hyperthermia. (See Nursing Care Related to "H.")
(6) Respiratory difficulties. (See Nursing Care Related to "B.")
(7) Changes in his sensory and motor consciousness. (See, also, Nursing Care Related to "N" and "O.")

6. When injury to the vertebral column has occurred (or is suspected),

A. The patient should preferably be kept in the position he is in until medical direction can be obtained.

B. If it is necessary to transport or adjust the position of the patient,

(1) Any flexion of the spine should be avoided.
(2) He may be placed on his back if the cervical region is involved.
(3) He may be placed on his abdomen if the thoracic or lumbar region is involved.

C. Medical orders concerning the movement or positioning of

the patient should be followed specifically (e.g. frequency of turning, use of special frames or braces).

D. Any support used for the trunk should be firm (e.g. use of special board under the mattress).

7. When there is injury to the bones of the thoracic cage,
   A. The chest wall should be supported (e.g. use of sandbags or strapping).
   B. The patient should be observed closely for respiratory difficulties.
   C. Activities involving the thorax or causing labored breathing should be restricted.
   D. Medical orders concerning the positioning of the patient, breathing exercises or exercise involving the upper extremities should be followed specifically.
8. When there is a weak area in the abdominal wall,
   A. It should be supported (e.g. with use of a binder), and this will be of particular importance during coughing, sneezing or vomiting.
   B. Certain kinds of exercise may be undesirable (e.g. descending stairs, stretching or heavy lifting).
   C. And there is herniation into the scrotum, the scrotum should be kept well-supported.
   D. The use of the abdominal muscles in lifting the body to a sitting position should be discouraged.
9. Women should be encouraged to have competent obstetrical care during pregnancy, labor, delivery and during the postpartum period.
10. When a patient has abnormal locomotor function (e.g. paralysis or tremors), adequate provision should be made for helping the patient to meet his physical needs.
11. Muscle relaxation may be promoted by:
    A. Massage.
    B. Positive relaxation exercises.
    C. Positioning.
    D. Heat.
    E. Elimination of irritating stimuli (e.g. pain, noise or bright light).

12. When muscle fatigue occurs,
    A. The muscles affected should be put at rest.
    B. Measures to improve circulation to the part may be used (e.g. contrast heat and cold).
13. When simple muscle spasm (cramping) occurs,
    A. The affected muscle may be carefully placed on stretch (e.g. spasm of the gastrocnemius may be relieved by dorsal flexion of the foot).
    B. Gentle massage of the muscle may be used.
    C. Heat may be applied.
14. When muscle spasm is severe and/or associated with central nervous system pathology (e.g. poliomyelitis),
    A. The muscles affected should be put at rest in the position of comfort.
    B. Anti-spasmodic drugs may be administered as ordered.
    C. Heat may be applied.
15. When muscle spasms recur frequently, this should be reported promptly.
16. When periarticular structures (e.g. ligaments, muscles or bursae) are inflamed, torn or stretched,
    A. The involved joint should be immobilized.
    B. Heat or cold may be used.
17. When fracture of a bone has occurred or is suspected, the immediate care should include either:
    A. Leaving the affected part in the position assumed until medical assistance is available or,
    B. If transportation is necessary, accomplishing it with the least possible amount of motion of the injured part.
       (1) The affected part should be splinted if possible.
          (a) A traction-type splint is preferable for the extremities.
          (b) Splinting of bones requires immobilization of the joints above and below the injury.
          (c) If the knee or elbow is injured and no traction is available, the full lengths of the articulating bones should be splinted in the position which has been assumed.

(2) If the hip is injured, movement of it should be avoided and the extremity affected should be allowed to remain in the position of comfort.

18. When a compound fracture of a bone has occurred, immediate care includes:
    A. The control of any bleeding. (See Nursing Care Related to "A.")
    B. Covering the wound.
    C. The application of a splint (not traction type) if transportation of the patient is necessary.
19. When there has been injury (including surgery) involving bone, muscle, joint or peripheral nerve, it is important that the following be known:
    A. The objective of any therapy being used (e.g. traction).
    B. The extent to which the patient may move or be moved.
    C. The positions in which the patient (or the injured part) may be placed.
20. When a patient has had traction applied
    A. And the objective is to immobilize and align a part,
       (1) The injured part should be maintained in the exact alignment in which it was placed by the physician.
       (2) The traction apparatus should be maintained as it has been arranged (e.g. weights and alignment of pulleys).
    B. And the objective is to stretch contracted muscles or to relieve pain,
       (1) The traction may be interrupted for nursing care as permitted by the physician.
       (2) Changes of position may be made as permitted by the physician.
21. If a patient in traction tends to be pulled toward the weights, counter-traction should be applied (preferably by elevating the end of the bed).
22. When internal skeletal fixation devices (e.g. pins or wires) are being used, the patient should be observed closely for signs and symptoms of local and/or systemic infection.
23. When traction or a cast has been applied,

A. The patient should be observed closely for signs and symptoms of:
   (1) Interference with circulation to the part. (See Nursing Care Related to "A.")
   (2) Bleeding.
   (3) Peripheral nerve damage (e.g. tingling, burning or numbness of part).

B. Any signs or symptoms related to the above should be reported promptly.

C. The body part extending beyond a cast or partially movable within a cast should be kept in the same alignment as the body parts which are held immovable by the cast.

D. The injured part should be supported in good alignment.

E. The injured extremity may be elevated as ordered.

F. The cast should be protected from dampness.

24. When a cast has been applied and circulation in the extremity is markedly decreased or there are signs of peripheral nerve damage and prompt medical assistance is not available (e.g. within minutes), the cast should be bivalved and the dressings underneath loosened.

25. When a patient has inflammation of a joint (e.g. rheumatoid arthritis),
   A. The body parts should be maintained in as normal alignment as possible. (The hands and feet should be kept in position of function.)
   B. The affected joint should be immobilized as ordered.
   C. Exercises involving the affected joint should be done as ordered.
      (1) The joint should be moved through complete range of motion up to the point of pain.
      (2) There should be opportunity for alternate contraction and relaxation of muscles.
      (3) If any exercise is followed by increased pain or swelling of the joint, this should be reported.
   D. The joint should be handled gently and kept well supported.
   E. Heat should be applied as ordered (e.g. hot packs, dry heat or paraffin baths).

F. Any signs of increasing limitations of motion or deformity should be reported.

PRINCIPLES OF ANATOMY AND PHYSIOLOGY UNDERLYING THE NURSING CARE

K. The muscular and skeletal systems provide a means of locomotion, support for body structures and protection for soft tissues.

General Facts Related to the Bony Skeleton

1. The skeleton is composed of a definite arrangement of bones joined together by ligaments, cartilage and muscles.
   A. The skeleton provides:
      (1) A framework for the body.
      (2) Protection for soft tissues.
      (3) A system of levers for locomotion.
   B. Each bone has a distinctive size and shape.
   C. The bones of the skeleton are joined to one another by connective tissue structures which permit varying degrees of movement between the adjoining bones.
      (1) The amount of motion permitted at an articulation depends upon the shapes of the adjoining bones and the arrangement of ligaments, tendons and muscles surrounding the joint.
         (a) Muscle tension interferes with joint motion.
         (b) Prolonged immobilization can cause joint stiffness and limitation in range of motion.
      (2) A freely movable joint has the following characteristics:
         (a) The contiguous bony surfaces are covered with hyaline cartilage.
         (b) A fibrous capsule surrounds the articulation.
         (c) Synovial membrane lines the capsule and is thought to secrete the lubricating synovial fluid.
         (d) Some joints may be divided by menisci.
      (3) A bursa is a small closed sac which contains a film of fluid and acts as a lubricating device. (Bursae may be found wherever tendons rub against resistant

structures, in some joint cavities and, subcutaneously, over joints which undergo acute flexion or over bones which are subject to considerable pressure.)

2. Bone is a plastic tissue composed of an organic portion which gives pliability and an inorganic portion which gives hardness and rigidity.
   A. The balance between the amount of organic and inorganic content changes with age.
      (1) The amount of inorganic substance increases with age, while the amount of organic substance decreases.
      (2) The long bones in children are largely cartilaginous and calcification is usually not complete until the eighteenth or twentieth year. (Usually the epiphyses do not close until this time, also.)
   B. Pressure, stresses and weight bearing can alter the shape and growth of bones.
   C. When bone is not functioning for locomotion over a prolonged period of time, there is some decalcification of the osseous tissue; this may result in an increased excretion of calcium in the urine.
   D. Hypocalcemia may cause the withdrawal of calcium from bones to raise the blood level of the calcium.
3. After severe injury to bone, there is hemorrhage, and granulation tissue is formed (called procallus). The granulation tissue becomes dense connective tissue, and then fibrocartilaginous tissue (callus) develops in the gap between the fragments. Ossification and calcification follow.
   A. Bony union of the fracture is accomplished when the new spongy bone invading the callus from the periosteum of the 2 fragments of the bone, makes contact and unites.
   B. The rate of bone healing decreases with age.

General Facts Related to the Voluntary Muscles and Neuromuscular Mechanism

1. All the movements of the body are brought about through the actions of muscles.
   A. Muscles are formed by groups of muscle fibers held together by connective tissue.

B. Muscles are firmly attached to bones by connective tissue.

2. Muscle tissue performs mechanical work by contracting; that is, by a shortening and thickening of its fibers.
   A. Muscle contractions occur as a result of complex oxidation-reduction reactions (involving carbohydrates) which occur in the muscle.
   B. Continuous or frequently repeated "all-out" contractions of a muscle or a long continued holding of a muscle in a state of contraction may cause injury to the muscle.
   C. Violent contractions may cause tearing, stretching or even rupture of muscles and their blood vessels.
   D. Muscle contraction is under nervous control.
      (1) Muscles are under more or less continuous nervous stimulation, and the rotational contractions of different groups of muscle fibers within the muscle result in tonus.
      (2) The myotatic (stretch) reflex is essential for maintaining skeletal muscle tone which in turn is essential for maintaining the normal condition of muscle fibers.
         (a) Atrophy and flaccidity occur in lower motor neuron lesions.
         (b) The tonus of the anti-gravity muscles (e.g. those of the jaw) is markedly decreased during sleep or when there is depression of the central nervous system (e.g. during general anesthesia).
         (c) The integrity of the higher centers (lying in the cortex and reticular formations) is essential for the maintenance of normal muscle tonus. These in turn are influenced by proprioceptive impulses arising within the muscle itself.
         (d) Tendon jerks are examples of myotatic reflexes.
         (e) Muscles which hold the body erect or are involved in locomotion lose their tone very rapidly during prolonged periods of inactivity.
      (3) Clonus is caused by the repeated synchronus activation of many motor units.
      (4) Tetany (prolonged contractions) is caused by the

continuous nervous stimulation of muscle groups. (Neuromuscular irritability is increased in hypocalcemia.)

(5) Change in position of any body part depends upon a constant series of nervous impulses mediated by efferent nerves which cause smooth coordinated contractions of the agonist muscles and relaxation of the antagonistic muscles involved.

3. Many areas of the cerebral cortex control motor function. (The major motor area concerned with voluntary movement is located just in front of the central fissure in the frontal lobe.)
4. Motor pathways pass directly or indirectly (through subcortical integration centers) to the medulla where up to 85 per cent of the fibers cross before entering the spinal cord.
5. The motor fibers pass down the spinal cord in several tracts and synapse with the lower motor neurons in the anterior horns of the spinal cord.
6. The individual muscles innervated by the motor nerves lie either approximately at the same level or below the level of origin of the lower motor neurons.
7. The spinal nerves which supply the upper and lower extremities, divide, recombine and divide again in complicated patterns to form 2 nerve plexuses.
   A. The brachial plexuses are located between the neck and the axilla in each shoulder, and the nerves supply all the muscles of the upper extremities.
   B. The lumbosacral plexuses are located in the lower back and the nerves supply all the muscles of the lower extremities.
8. The peripheral nerves are subject to injury through trauma, stretching or pressure; if traumatized, the part they supply is paralyzed and rendered insensitive. Nerves which run very superficially in the extremities include the peroneal (in the popliteal space), the ulnar (along medial upper arm and down the ulna side of the forearm), the radial (around the back of the humerus and down the radial side of the forearm) and the sciatic (in hip and down the back of the thigh).

9. The functions of the cerebellum are concerned with equilibrium, postural reflexes, regulation of muscle tone and coordination of voluntary movement.
10. Proprioceptors, located in the skeletal muscles, tendons and joints, are sensitive to pressure or stretch and transmit impulses to the brain via the posterior columns of the spinal cord.
    A. These impulses provide information about movements and the position of the limbs and are important for muscular coordination.
    B. The conscious interpretation of the impulses takes place in the temporal and parietal lobes of the cerebral cortex.
11. Injury to the motor neurons may result in:
    A. Flaccid or spastic paralysis.
    B. Depressed or exaggerated reflexes.
    C. Abnormal motor activity.
        (1) Involuntary movements.
        (2) Muscular rigidity.
        (3) Muscular incoordination.
        (4) Ataxia.
        (5) Difficulty with postural adjustments.
12. Irritation of the meninges often results in nuchal rigidity.
13. Flexor reflexes play an important role in the abrupt withdrawal of an injured part from the source of hurt.
    A. The flexor reflex involves, basically:
        (1) Peripheral sensory receptors for pain.
        (2) Internuncial nerves in the spinal cord.
        (3) Peripheral motor nerves.
    B. Subcortical centers in the midbrain, thalamus and/or spinal cord may also be involved in flexor reflexes.
14. Following spinal transection, all somatic and autonomic reflexes may be abolished for some time.
15. In deep anesthesia many reflexes are completely abolished.
16. There are reflex mechanism governing the orientation of the head in space, the relation of the head to the trunk and the appropriate adjustments of the limbs to the position of the head.

A. Sensory nerve endings in the inner ear, retina and in the skeletal muscles, tendons and joints receive stimuli.
B. Impulses are transmitted to the spinal cord, midbrain and cerebellum.
C. Motor nerves cause appropriate postural adjustments.

Specific Facts about Bones, Muscles and Joints Concerned Primarily with Locomotion

1. The bones of the upper extremity include those of the shoulder girdle (clavicle and scapula), the upper arm (humerus), the lower arm (radius and ulna), the wrist (8 carpal bones) and the hand (5 metacarpal bones and 14 phalanges).
2. The shoulder joint, formed by the articulation of the head of the humerus with the scapula, is of the ball and socket type.
   A. The socket is shallow.
   B. The ligaments surrounding the joint are relatively loose.
   C. The shoulder joint allows movement of the humerus in all directions.
   D. The scapula is connected to the trunk by muscles only.
3. Muscles which originate on the trunk and insert on the shoulder girdle (acting singly or in combinations) act to adduct, abduct, elevate, depress and to rotate the shoulder girdle.
4. Muscles which originate on the trunk and shoulder girdle and insert on the humerus (acting singly or in combinations) act to adduct, abduct, flex, extend and to rotate the humerus.
5. The elbow joint comprises 3 different portions: the joints between the ulna and humerus, the radius and humerus, and the radius and the ulna.
   A. The joint between the ulna and the humerus is a simple hinge joint.
   B. Muscles which originate on the shoulder girdle and/or the humerus and insert on the radius or ulna act to flex and to extend the forearm.
   C. Muscles which originate and insert on the ulna and radius act to supinate and to pronate the forearm.

6. The wrist joint proper formed by the articulations of several carpal bones and the distal end of the radius, is of the gliding type.
   A. Muscles of the posterior aspect of the forearm act to extend the hand.
   B. Muscles of the anterior aspect of the forearm act to flex the hand.
   C. The flexors and extensors acting in different groupings also abduct, adduct and circumduct the hand.
7. The joints between the metacarpal and carpal bones are of the gliding type and have limited motion with the exception of the first metacarpal which is a saddle joint and allows for abduction, adduction, circumduction and opposition of the thumb.
8. The joints between the metacarpal and phalangeal bones are of the condyloid type and allow flexion, extension, limited abduction and adduction and circumduction of the fingers.
9. The joints between the phalanges of each digit are of the hinge type and allow for flexion and extension.
10. The vertebral column is composed of individual vertebrae, the bodies of which are separated by fibro-cartilaginous discs and all of which are bound together by numerous ligaments which pass from one bone to another.
   A. The intervertebral discs absorb shock and permit a slight degree of movement.
   B. The vertebral column articulates with the skull and with the iliac bones of the pelvic girdle.
11. At birth and until a baby is able to hold up his head, the primary curve of the vertebral column is posteriorly convex. After the baby's muscles have developed enough so that he can hold up his head and stand and walk, the secondary curves of the vertebral column appear.
   A. The cervical curve is anteriorly convex.
   B. The thoracic curve is posteriorly convex.
   C. The lumbar curve is anteriorly convex.
   D. The natural curves of the vertebral column give resilience and help to absorb shock.

   E. The natural curves may be changed by prolonged postural changes, variations in walking and pregnancy.
   F. In walking or sitting the pelvic girdle normally provides support for the vertebral column.

12. Muscles of the back which essentially attach vertebrae to vertebrae or vertebrae to ribs act to extend the spine and assist in rotation of the spine. (These muscles are fixator muscles and are arranged primarily for the purpose of support, not for the performance of work.)
13. Muscles which originate on the pelvic girdle and insert on the ribs act to flex the spine.
14. Muscles which originate on the vertebrae or shoulder girdle and insert on the posterior skull act to extend the head.
15. Muscles which originate on the temporal bone or cervical vertebrae and insert on the clavicle or rib cage act to flex the head.
16. The bones of the lower extremity include those of the pelvic girdle (innominate bones, sacrum and coccyx), the thigh (femur), the leg (tibia and fibula), the ankle (7 tarsal bones) and the foot (5 metatarsal bones and 14 phalanges).
    A. The innominate bones articulate anteriorly at the symphysis pubis.
    B. During pregnancy a hormone causes some relaxation of the ligaments of the pelvic girdle.
17. The hip joint, formed by the articulation of the head of the femur fitting into the acetabulum of the innominate bone, is of the ball and socket type.
18. Muscles which originate on the vertebrae or pelvic girdle and insert on the femur (acting singly or in combinations) act to flex, extend, abduct, adduct or to rotate the femur.
19. The knee joint, formed by the articulation of the distal femur and the tibia, is both condyloid and gliding.
    A. The knee movements are closely related to movements of the hip joint.
    B. The patella is a flat bone located in the tendon on the quadriceps femoris in front of the knee joint and articulates with the femur. (It helps to protect the knee joint, especially in kneeling.)

C. Menisci lie between the tibia and the femur and help to adapt the surfaces of these bones and to obviate jars.

20. Muscles which originate on the pelvic girdle or femur and insert on the tibia (acting singly or in combinations) act to extend, flex and, in certain positions, to rotate (medially and laterally) the lower leg.
21. The ankle joint, formed by the articulation of the distal ends of the tibia and fibula and one of the tarsal bones is both hinge and condyloid in type.
   A. Muscles which originate on the tibia and fibula and insert on the medial or lateral aspects of the tarsal or metatarsal bones act either to invert or evert the foot.
   B. Muscles which originate on the anterior aspects of the tibia and fibula and insert on the tarsal bones act to dorsiflex the foot.
   C. Muscles which originate on the posterior aspects of the femur, tibia and fibula and insert on the tarsal bones act to plantar-flex the foot. (The major muscles which act to plantar-flex the foot insert in the tendon of Achilles.)
22. The tarsal and metatarsal articulations allow limited gliding motions.
23. The metatarsal and phalangeal articulations allow some flexion, extension, abduction and adduction.
24. The interphalangeal joints permit flexion and limited extension.
25. The foot has a longitudinal arch and a series of transverse arches formed by the arrangement of the tarsal and metatarsal bones and the ligaments which bind them together. (When the body is raised on the ball of one foot, the stress on the longitudinal arch is increased fourfold.)

Facts Related to Posture

1. Good posture may be defined as the good anatomical relationships of the body parts to each other when the body is in different positions.
   A. The alignment of the body parts should be balanced and there should not be undue muscle tension or strain.

B. Correct body posture exists when the muscular forces required to balance torques produced by the weights of various parts of the body are at a minimum.

2. A good lying posture in the dorsal recumbent position is the closest as is possible to the good standing posture.
3. A good lying posture in the supine position is the closest as is possible to the good standing posture with the head turned to the side.
4. A good lying posture in the side-lying postion is an approximation of a good sitting posture.
5. The position of function for the hand is similar to that position used in gripping a ball.
6. The position of function for the foot is that position which is desirable in good standing posture.

Specific Facts about Bones and Muscles Which Protect and Support Underlying Soft Tissues

1. The bony structures which protect soft tissue include the skull, vertebral column, rib cage, and pelvic girdle.
2. The bones of the skull protect the contents of the cranium, including the brain and the meninges, blood vessels and the cerebrospinal fluid.
   A. Some of the bones of the skull (frontal, parietal, temporal, and occipital) are united in suture lines (immovable joints).
   B. The suture lines are not united at birth and there are unossified areas between the bones.
      (1) The anterior fontanel lies between the 2 parietal and frontal bones and normally closes within 1½ years.
      (2) The posterior fontanel lies between the 2 parietal and the occipital bones and normally closes within 6 months.
3. The vertebrae protect the contents of the neural canal.
   A. The neural canal, containing the spinal cord, meninges, and spinal fluid, is formed by the bodies and processes of the vertebrae.
   B. Spinal nerves emerge from the neural canal through the

intervertebral foramina which are posterior to the bodies of the vertebrae and between the bases of successive arches.

4. The thoracic cage is composed of the 12 thoracic vertebrae which articulate with the 12 pairs of ribs some of which, in turn, articulate with the sternum and the clavicle.
   A. Within the thoracic cage lie the lungs, the heart and the great vessels.
   B. Movement of the ribs by costal muscles plays an important role in breathing.
   C. The diaphragm, which plays an important role in breathing, originates in part on the ribs and sternum.
5. The muscles of the abdominal wall are flat muscles which extend from the pelvic girdle or lumbodorsal fascia to the costal cartilages and they help to support and protect the abdominal and pelvic viscera.
   A. The separated rectus abdominis muscles extend from the pubes to the anterior rib cage and are relatively weak muscles. (The umbilicus lies between the separated rectus muscles and transmits the umbilical cord in the unborn child.)
   B. The inguinal canal (which transmits the spermatic cord in the male and the round ligament in the female) runs through the lower portion of the abdominal muscles above the inguinal ligament. It has 2 openings: a superficial one in the external oblique close to the body of the pubis and a deep opening which lies more laterally and opens into the abdominal cavity.
   C. The abdominal muscles contract and exert pressure against the abdominal viscera in:
      (1) Forced expiration.
      (2) Coughing.
      (3) Vomiting.
      (4) Voluntary compression during such processes as micturition and defecation.
      (5) Flexion of the vertebral column.
      (6) Lifting legs when lying in horizontal position.

(7) Lifting heavy objects.

D. The abdominal muscles are stretched in pregnancy and in activities such as reaching high above the head and descending stairs.

6. The muscles of the pelvic floor support part of the weight of the abdominal and pelvic viscera.
   A. These muscles include the paired levator ani and coccygeus muscles.
   B. During childbirth these muscles are stretched and may be torn.

PRINCIPLES OF PHYSICS UNDERLYING THE NURSING CARE

K. The muscular and skeletal systems provide a means of locomotion, support for body structures and protection for soft tissues.

1. Force is that which changes or tends to change the linear motion of a body, and the motion is in the same direction as the force.
2. Work is done by a force if the force is allowed to act through a distance.
3. Torque is that which changes or tends to change the rotary motion of a body.
4. Gravitation is the force of attraction between 2 objects (e.g. the earth and an object on or near the earth).
   A. The center of gravity of a body is the point where the whole weight of a body may be considered to be concentrated. (The center of gravity in the human body is located at a point approximately 0.57 of the height of the body.)
   B. Because of gravitational pull, more force is usually required to lift a heavy object than to push or pull it along a smooth surface.
5. A body is said to be unstable if a slight tipping of the object raises its center of gravity.
   A. A vertical line drawn downward from the center of gravity

of a body in stable equilibrium will fall within the base of support. (Increasing the base of support will increase stability.)

B. In general, a change in the position of the center of gravity upsets equilibrium and, for equilibrium to be regained, changes must be made in forces and/or torques acting on the object (e.g. in standing, when there is a forward shift in the center of gravity, the muscles of the back must exert more pull to maintain body balance).

6. When a body is in equilibrium,
   A. The resultant of all forces acting on the body equals zero, and
   B. The resultant of all torques acting at any axis must equal zero.
7. Within the elastic limit, the stress is proportional to the strain. (Hooke's Law)
   A. If the elastic limit of an object is exceeded, the object is either permanently distorted or broken.
   B. Types of stress which may produce characteristic injuries in the body are tension, compression, twisting and bending.
8. A lever is a simple machine comprising a rigid bar which moves about a fulcrum (or fixed axis). Keeping lever arms short decreases the torque produced by a given load.

PRINCIPLES OF CHEMISTRY UNDERLYING THE NURSING CARE

K. The muscular and skeletal systems provide a means of locomotion, support for body structures and protection for soft tissues.

1. Plaster of Paris powder combines with water to form a solid mass of large crystals of gypsum, which occupy a larger volume than the original powder and water. (The crystals of gypsum are slightly soluble in water so that plaster casts can be weakened by being wet.)
2. Some plastic materials used for casts shrink as they dry.

Section L: Nursing Care and Science Principles Related to the Skin and Mucous Membranes.

L. Unbroken healthy skin and mucous membranes serve as first lines of defense against harmful agents.

NURSING CARE

1. All patients should be observed for signs and symptoms of injury to the skin and these should be reported. This is of particular importance when there is:
   A. Skin disease or a condition which affects the skin.
   B. A patient with a known delicate or sensitive skin.
   C. Peripheral circulatory disease.
   D. Prolonged bedrest, especially if the patient is overweight, emaciated or elderly.
   E. Decreased sensitivity to pain and temperature.
   F. Inability to move.
   G. Generalized or dependent edema.
   H. Incontinence or drainage onto the skin.
   I. Equipment used on or through the skin (e.g. casts or skeletal traction devices).
   J. Application of physical or chemical agents to the skin.
2. Signs and symptoms of injury (or possible injury) to the skin may include:
   A. Color changes.
   B. Lesions (e.g. vesicles, papules or excoriations).
   C. Maceration.
   D. Corns, calluses.
   E. Scaling (e.g. dandruff).

- F. Bleeding.
- G. Itching
- H. Edema.

3. The skin should be protected from mechanical injury by:
   - A. The reduction of friction (e.g. proper-fitting shoes, secure bandages or use of caution when moving patient in bed).
   - B. The use of appropriate methods to remove substances adhered to the skin.
   - C. The avoidance of cutting the skin with sharp objects (e.g. care in shaving or padding edges of casts).
   - D. The avoidance of breaking blisters or squeezing pimples.
   - E. The use of treatments and medications as ordered to relieve itching. (See Nursing Care Related to "N.")
   - F. The discouragement of scratching (e.g. use of restraint or proper care of hands and nails).
   - G. The discouragement of the use of irritating substances on the skin (e.g. some beautifying agents).
   - H. The avoidance of pressure, especially over bony prominences or ears.
4. The skin should be protected from physical injury by:
   - A. The use of caution when administering treatments involving heat.
     - (1) Great caution should be observed when administering treatments involving temperature change (hot or cold) to patients who:
       - (a) Have a peripheral circulatory problem (e.g. atherosclerosis, Buerger's disease, frostbite or edema).
       - (b) Have loss of sensation (e.g. cordotomy, peripheral nerve damage or coma).
       - (c) Have little subcutaneous tissue (or when areas of the body having little subcutaneous tissue are involved).
       - (d) Are unable to move.
       - (e) Are having prolonged periods of therapy involving heat or cold.
     - (2) The temperature of hot water used in treatments involving heat should be measured with a thermometer.

(An exception is water used externally for bathing or external irrigations; in this case, the temperature may be tested on the inner aspect of the arm or on an area of the patient's skin which has a lesser degree of sensitivity.

(3) If a marked degree of hyperemia and/or discomfort occurs during the application of heat, the treatment should be temporarily discontinued or less heat used.

B. The use of caution when applying cold for prolonged periods of time.

C. The use of caution in length and degree of exposure to ultra-violet rays and infra-red rays.

D. The provision for occasional drying of the skin when wet packs or soaks are used for a prolonged time.

E. The use of emollients as necessary.

F. The avoidance of drying agents (e.g. alcohol) when the skin is abnormally dry.

G. The use of caution when administering fluids subcutaneously.

(1) The subcutaneous injections of relatively large amounts of fluid (hypodermoclysis) should be done slowly and the rate of flow should be regulated according to the absorption rate.

(2) The hypodermic injection of a drug should be administered intramuscularly rather than subcutaneously when an amount more than 1 cc. is to be given. (Exceptions are insulin and other drugs which are specifically ordered to be administered subcutaneously. In these cases multiple injections may have to be made.)

5. The skin should be protected from chemical injury by:

A. The removal of irritating body secretions.

B. The avoidance of injurious chemicals on or in the skin (e.g. caution in the use of disinfectant solutions, adhesive tape, deodorants or in administration of intravenous injections).

C. The use of protectives as necessary on the normal, unbroken skin.

D. The avoidance of:
   (1) The use of strongly alkaline soaps.
   (2) Overuse of soap or detergents.

6. The skin should be protected from microbial injury by preventing mechanical, physical or chemical injury to it.
7. When injury to the skin has occurred,
   A. Clean or aseptic technique should be used in the care of the wound.
   B. Tension around the wound should be avoided.
   C. Caution should be used in the care of the injured skin (e.g. gentleness in removal of adhered dressings).
   D. Injured tissue or exposed underlying tissues should be protected from harmful chemical or physical agents.
      (1) Only mild, non-irritating solutions should be used for cleaning wound (e.g. physiological saline solution or dilute mild soap solution).
      (2) No antiseptic solution or disinfectant should be applied to injured tissue without medical orders.
      (3) Caution should be used in the application of heat or cold to injured tissue.
   E. The area should be observed for signs of infection. (See Nursing Care Related to "M.")
   F. The area should be observed for the process of healing and abnormalities should be reported.
8. When there is skin disease associated with emotional disturbances, possible causative psychological factors should be recognized and supportive care should be given as indicated.
9. All patients should be observed for signs and symptoms of injury to mucous membranes and these should be reported. This is of particular importance when there is:
   A. Disease or surgical condition involving the respiratory, digestive or genito-urinary tract.
   B. Tubes inserted into body cavities.
   C. Problem of dehydration.
   D. Condition in which the dietary oral intake is restricted.
10. Reportable signs and symptoms of injury (or possible injury) to mucous membrane may include:
    A. Color changes.

B. Lesions (e.g. ulcerations).
C. Excessive or decreased production of mucous or saliva.
D. Bleeding.
E. Discomfort.
F. Edema.

11. Mucous membranes should be protected from mechanical injury by:
    A. The use of appropriate lubricants in performing treatments.
    B. The insertion of tubes and instruments into body cavities gently and in the correct directions.
    C. The use of smooth objects in performing treatments.
    D. The use of tubes of proper size for insertion into body cavities.
    E. The avoidance of harsh purgatives or high roughage foods.
    F. The encouragement of the proper mastication of foods.
    G. The use of caution in suctioning the respiratory tract (e.g. avoidance of the over-use or use of too strong suction).
    H. The humidification of air or oxygen as necessary. (Mouth breathing should be discouraged.)
    I. The proper cleansing and moistening of the nose, mouth or trachea (latter, if tracheotomy exists).
    J. The encouragement of fluid intake.
12. Mucous membranes should be protected from physical injury by the use of caution in treatments involving heat.
    A. A thermometer should be used to check the temperature of solutions used in irrigations.
    B. Gargles and throat irrigation solutions may be as hot as tolerated comfortably—about 120° F.
13. Mucous membranes should be protected from chemical injury by:
    A. The avoidance of strong chemicals or concentrated solutions for treatments (e.g. strong soap solutions for enemas or concentrated antiseptic solutions for irrigations).
    B. The use of small feedings of milk and/or cream when there are symptoms of minor irritation of a gastric or duodenal ulcer or heartburn.

   C. Proper cleansing of the external genitalia.
14. Mucous membranes should be protected from microbial injury by:
   A. The prevention of mechanical, physical or chemical injury to them.
   B. The discouragement of frequent vaginal irrigations or irrigations with antiseptic solutions (unless ordered by physician).
15. When there is a possibility of chemical injury to the mucous membrane lining of the stomach or upper small intestine (e.g. due to gastric secretions), possible causative psychological factors should be recognized and supportive care should be given as indicated.
16. When mucous membrane has been injured,
   A. Clean or aseptic technique should be used in treatments.
   B. Gentleness should be used in the care of the injured tissue.
   C. Strong chemicals should not be used for treatments.
      (1) Physiological saline solution or water may be used.
      (2) Proper dilutions of irrigating solutions should be prepared.
      (3) No antiseptic nor disinfectant drugs should be applied to the wound without medical orders.
   D. The area should be observed for signs of infection (as possible).
   E. The area should be observed for the process of healing (as possible).

PRINCIPLES OF ANATOMY AND PHYSIOLOGY UNDERLYING THE NURSING CARE

L. Unbroken healthy skin and mucous membranes serve as first lines of defense against harmful agents.

Facts Related to the Skin

1. Skin envelops the entire surface of the body, and its epithelium is continuous with the epithelium of the external orifices of the digestive, respiratory and genito-urinary tracts.

2. The skin is rich in cutaneous sensory nerves for pain, touch or pressure, heat and cold.
3. The dermis of the skin has many blood vessels, but the epidermis is avascular, nourished by circulating tissue fluid only.
4. The skin may be dry or moist, rough or smooth depending upon the amount and nature of keratinized epidermis and the amount and nature of the secretions of the cutaneous glands.
   A. Sebum, an oily secretion produced by the sebaceous glands, keeps the skin soft and supple and prevents passage of water through the skin. (There is decreased sebum production in old age.)
   B. Continuous rubbing and pressure causes great thickening of the epidermis.
5. The color of the skin varies with the vascularity.
   A. Intense scarlet indicates increased blood flow in dilated vessels.
   B. Pallor or light pink color indicates moderate-sized or somewhat constricted superficial vessels.
   C. Ashen type of cyanosis indicates slowed cutaneous flow and constricted superficial vessels.
6. The temperature of the skin depends largely upon the amount and rate of blood flow through its vessels.
7. Skin is firm over bony prominences and may be flaccid over soft parts.
8. Individual skins vary in their resistance to injury. Factors which affect resistance include:
   A. The general health of the cells (e.g. circulation or nutrition).
   B. The amount of subcutaneous tissue. (Very much or very little subcutaneous tissue tends to decrease resistance.)
   C. The degree of pigmentation (in relation to ultra-violet rays).
9. The cutaneous vascular responses to injury include:
   A. The white reaction (capillary constriction).
   B. The red reaction (local vasodilation).
   C. The wheal (local edema). (When fluid collects between the layers of epidermis, a blister results.)

10. Normal physiologic response to externally applied heat or cold depends upon:
    A. Normal sensory perception.
    B. Normal vasomotor activity of the peripheral arterioles.
11. Prolonged stimulation by cold may cause a decrease of sensation in the area affected, due both to a decrease in the circulation and in the metabolic rate.
12. Prolonged stimulation by heat may cause:
    A. A decrease in the sensation (adaptation).
    B. Prolonged hyperemia.
13. Sweat glands in the axilla, groin and about the external genitalia are influenced by emotions and increased secretion may result in local eruptions and itching.
14. The scratch reflex is initiated by irritation of sensory receptors in the skin and involves, basically:
    A. Sensory and motor pathways in the cord.
    B. Sub-cortical centers in the midbrain and thalamus.
    C. Peripheral motor nerves.

Facts Related to Mucous Membrane

1. The respiratory, gastro-intestinal and genito-urinary tracts are lined with mucous membrane.
2. Mucous membrane is delicate.
3. Glandular cells in the mucosa or submucosa produce small amounts of mucus which:
    A. Keep the membrane surface moist.
    B. Serve as a lubricant.
    C. Act as a protectant (against acid and enzymes) of the cells lining the gastro-intestinal tract.
4. Emotions have a profound effect upon the vascularity of the mucosa of the stomach and upper small intestine.
5. Saliva and the process of mastication of food helps to keep the mucous membrane of the mouth and throat moist and clean.
6. Irritation of mucous membrane generally causes increased production of mucus, but may cause a reduction in amount.
7. The pH of the vaginal secretions is normally slightly acidic.

FACTS RELATED TO BOTH THE SKIN AND MUCOUS MEMBRANE

1. The continuity of the skin or mucous membrane may be broken by:
   A. Mechanical means (e.g. cutting or scraping).
   B. Physical means (e.g. burns due to heat or radiation).
   C. Chemical means (e.g. acids).
   D. Disease processes (e.g. communicable diseases which involve skin lesions).
2. Some of the body fluids contain chemicals or may be decomposed by bacteria to release chemicals which are irritating to the skin and mucous membranes (e.g. urine, sweat, colostrum, exudates or digestive juices).
3. Following injury to the skin or mucous membrane,
   A. There is usually bleeding (will depend upon extent of injury) followed by the formation of a clot.
   B. Tissue fluid is lost.
   C. Normally, granulation tissue develops and this eventually becomes scar tissue.
4. The rate and quality of wound healing depend upon many factors, including:
   A. The approximation of wound edges.
   B. The presence of infection in the wound.
   C. The presence of foreign material in the wound.
   D. Any trauma of the wound and surrounding tissues.
   E. Circulation of the affected part.
   F. General health of the patient (e.g. nutritional state).
   G. Age of the patient. (Healing occurs more rapidly in the young.)

PRINCIPLES OF PHYSICS UNDERLYING THE NURSING CARE

L. Unbroken healthy skin and mucous membranes serve as first lines of defense against harmful agents.

1. Friction is that force which opposes motion between 2 contacting surfaces.

A. Friction is caused by surface irregularities.
B. Friction may be decreased by decreasing the irregularities (e.g. through smoothing the surfaces or separating the surfaces with lubrication).

PRINCIPLES OF CHEMISTRY UNDERLYING THE NURSING CARE

L. Unbroken healthy skin and mucous membranes serve as first lines of defense against harmful agents.

1. An acid may be defined as a compound which gives hydrogen ions (or hydronium ions) in solution.
2. A base may be defined as a compound which yields hydroxyl ions in solutions.
3. The degree to which ionization to hydronium or hydroxyl ions occurs may be said to determine the strength of the acid or base. (Ammonia in a water solution is a fairly strong base.)
4. Surface tension of water may be decreased by soap and detergents.
   A. Soaps are metallic salts of fatty acids and, in aqueous solution, are slightly basic.
   B. Synthetic detergents can be more efficient than soap in lowering surface tension.
   C. The lowering of surface tension aids in the emulsification of lipids.
5. Polar liquids (e.g. water) tend to dissolve polar substances (e.g. inorganic salts) more readily than non-polar substances.
6. Non-polar liquids (e.g. ether, carbon disulfide or carbon tetrachloride) tend to dissolve non-polar substances (e.g. lipids) more readily than polar substances.

Section M: Nursing Care and Science Principles Related to the White Blood Cells and Antibodies.

M. The body is able to produce cellular elements and specific chemical substances which serve to protect the body against harmful agents.

NURSING CARE

1. All patients should be observed for symptoms of infection and these should be reported. This is of particular importance when the patient:
   A. Is an infant or young child.
   B. Is elderly.
   C. Has a condition in which there is a decrease in the number of mature leukocytes (e.g. leukemia).
   D. Has been exposed to a communicable disease to which he is not immune.
   E. Has a broken skin or mucous membrane (e.g. surgical wounds, burns or intrinsic skeletal fixation devices for fractured bones).
2. Reportable signs and symptoms of inflammations and/or infection may include:
   A. Fever with associated symptoms. (See Nursing Care Related to "H.")
   B. Cardinal symptoms of inflammation (pain, swelling, heat, redness and loss of function).
   C. Swelling and tenderness of lymph glands near the infected area.
   D. Discomfort in the normal body functions (e.g. swallowing or voiding).

E. Appearance of pus (e.g. wounds, eyes, ears or urine).
F. Red lines in the skin extending up an extremity.
G. Skin lesions (e.g. macules or pustules).

3. All patients should be protected from microbial injury. (See Nursing Care Related to "The Prevention of Microbial Injury.")
4. Special precautions should be taken to protect patients with defective body defenses (e.g. leukemia) from any type of physical injury and local or generalized infection.
5. When there is a local superficial inflammation and/or infection,
   A. Warm applications may be used.
   B. The area adjacent to the inflamed or infected area should not be injured (e.g. pimples should not be squeezed).
6. When there is drainage of material from an infected part (e.g. an infected middle ear), drainage may be promoted by positioning of the patient.
7. When local tissue edema (e.g. due to injury or allergic response) is beginning, cold applications may be used.
8. All patients should be observed for symptoms of allergy, and these should be reported. This is of particular importance when the patient:
   A. Has a history of hypersensitivity.
   B. Is receiving substances which are likely to cause allergic responses (e.g. transfusions, sera or drugs).
9. Reportable signs and symptoms of hypersensitivity may include:
   A. A rapid fall in blood pressure with associated symptoms. (See Nursing Care Related to "A.")
   B. Symptoms of obstructed airway. (See Nursing Care Related to "B.")
   C. Skin lesions.
      (1) Rash.
      (2) Urticaria.
      (3) Scaling.
   D. Hyperemia.
   E. Itching.
   F. Vomiting or diarrhea.

   G. Severe headache.
   H. Reddened, tearing eyes and puffy eyelids.
   I. Excessive mucus production in the respiratory tract.
   J. Pain in the joints.
10. Any known sensitivities to various substances (e.g. drugs or food) should be ascertained from the patient or his family, and the patient should be protected from contact with these substances.
11. When allergies are known to exist, medical orders may be sought concerning any immediate treatment of undesirable physiologic reactions.
12. When substances known to cause allergic responses relatively frequently are to be administered,
   A. Test doses may be used (e.g. tetanus antitoxin).
   B. Epinephrine and equipment for its administration should be kept in readiness.
13. When a patient has an allergic reaction following the administration of a particular drug, the doctor should be notified promptly and a repeated administration of the same drug should be avoided until further orders are received.
14. When a patient develops urticaria while receiving a blood transfusion, the rate of blood flow should be slowed and the physician notified of the symptom promptly.

PRINCIPLES OF ANATOMY AND PHYSIOLOGY UNDERLYING THE NURSING CARE

M. The body is able to produce cellular elements and specific chemical substances which serve to protect the body against harmful agents.

Facts Pertaining to White Blood Cells

1. The prime function of white blood cells is a protective one.
   A. Immature leukocytes are unable to function efficiently.
   B. Lymphocytes are associated with the inflammatory process.
   C. Monocytes and neutrophils phagocytize micro-organisms and debris.

D. All three help to isolate an infected area from neighboring healthy tissue.
E. Pus is composed largely of dead leukocytes along with living and dead micro-organisms.

2. There are normally 5000 to 9000 mature leukocytes per cubic millimeter of blood.
   A. Approximately 20 per cent are lymphocytes and 60 to 70 per cent are neutrophils.
   B. Tissue damage may result in leukocytosis.
3. Lymphocytes are formed in lymphoid tissue (e.g. spleen and lymph glands) and may be found in these organs in various stages of development. (Normally, they mature before entering the general circulation.)
4. Lymph glands are found at intervals along lymph vessels and have the functions of producing lymphocytes and of filtering out and destroying foreign bodies, including bacteria.
   A. Lymph ultimately empties into the systemic circulation by way of the right and left subclavian veins.
   B. Inflamed lymph vessels appear as fine red lines in the skin.
   C. The major groups of lymph glands which may be palpated easily or are noticeably tender when enlarged are those in:
      (1) The neck.
      (2) The axilla.
      (3) The groin.
   D. Lymph glands may become enlarged and tender when they have been infected by septic materials from regions which the lymphatic vessels drain.
   E. Enlargement of the tonsils may cause difficulty with swallowing.
   F. Enlargement of the adenoids may cause difficulty with nasal breathing.
5. Neutrophils develop in myeloid tissue and normally mature before entering the circulation. (Precursors of mature neutrophils are myelocytes.)

Facts Pertaining to the Inflammatory Process

1. The inflammatory response of tissues to injury includes:
   A. Vasodilatation in the affected part with an increased blood flow.
   B. Increased capillary permeability.
   C. Increased number of white blood cells at the site of injury.

Facts Pertaining to Antibodies

1. The function of antibodies is to protect the body cells from harmful antigens.
2. An antibody is a specific substance produced in the cells of the spleen, liver, lymph nodes, bone marrow and probably in other tissues from portions of gamma globulin, in response to the introduction of a specific antigen.
   A. Antibodies react with antigens in various ways to prevent harmful effects of the antigens.
   B. Any foreign material which may be introduced into the body may act as an antigen.
      (1) Foreign materials may be inhaled, ingested, injected or in simple contact with the body surface.
      (2) Physical agents also may act as antigens.
   C. Some antibodies remain in the tissues while others circulate in the blood.
   D. Antibodies pass from the mother to the baby in the placenta or through the milk.
   E. In hypersensitivity (or allergy) the antigen-antibody reaction produces undesirable physiological responses.
      (1) Histamine, formed in the tissues during allergic reactions, may cause:
         (a) Vasodilatation (local and/or generalized) which may be accompanied by edema.
         (b) Skin lesions.
         (c) Itching.
         (d) Tearing.
         (e) Bronchiolar constriction.
         (f) Excessive mucus production.

(g) Vomiting or diarrhea.
(h) Bleeding from mucous membrane.

(2) The severity of an allergic response depends upon the degree of sensitivity of the individual (the amount of antibodies produced) and the amount of the antigen introduced.

(3) Allergic response may be so severe as to threaten life.

PRINCIPLES OF PHYSICS UNDERLYING THE NURSING CARE

M. The body is able to produce cellular elements and specific chemical substances which serve to protect the body against harmful agents.

1. Gravitation is the force of attraction between 2 objects (e.g. the earth and an object on or near the earth).

Section N: Nursing Care and Science Principles Related to Physical Discomfort.

N. Sensations of physical discomfort may indicate injury or threat of injury to the body.

NURSING CARE

1. All patients should be observed for signs and symptoms of physical discomforts and these should be reported in detail.
   A. Patients should be observed closely for physical discomforts commonly associated with their conditions or with complications common to their conditions.
   B. Patients should be encouraged to report and discuss any physical discomforts. (Provision should be made for adequate means of communication.)
   C. Precise and complete information about physical discomforts should be sought persistently. This includes:
      (1) Localization of the discomfort.
      (2) Time of occurrence.
      (3) Frequency of occurrence.
      (4) Description of the type of discomfort.
   D. Evaluation of a patient's discomfort should be made by objectively interpreting all significant data. Such data may include:
      (1) The diagnosis of the patient and complaints commonly associated with his condition.
      (2) Complaints associated with complications common with his condition.
      (3) Severity and duration of the symptom.
      (4) Type of therapy he is receiving (e.g. drugs, surgery or treatments) together with normal and abnormal reactions to this therapy.

(5) General physical condition of the patient.
(6) Emotional status of the patient.
(7) Pain threshold of the patient.
(8) Age of the patient.
(9) Environmental factors (e.g. ward activities or ventilation).

E. The relative significance of the physical discomfort determines to whom and how promptly the symptom should be reported.
(1) Any sudden new pain or tenderness should be reported promptly.
(2) Any severe discomfort should be reported promptly.
(3) Discomfort which cannot be alleviated by nursing measures should be reported promptly.
(4) Pain associated with skeletal fixation devices such as casts or traction should be investigated and reported promptly.

F. A patient's reaction to physical discomfort may help in determining his level of consciousness.

2. Signs and symptoms of physical discomfort may include:
A. Vocalization, crying, moaning, or unusual quietness.
B. Increased muscular tension.
C. Pulse and blood pressure changes.
D. Skin color changes, changes in skin temperature.
E. Changes in facial expression (e.g. grimacing).
F. Breathing changes (e.g. hyperventilation).
G. Sweating.
H. Unusual postures (e.g. knees drawn up to abdomen).
I. Nausea and vomiting, anorexia.
J. Excessive salivation.
K. Restlessness, sleeplessness,
L. Behavioral changes (e.g. increased irritability).
M. Scratching or rubbing.
N. Frequency of urination.
O. Withdrawal from any pain-causing stimulus.

3. In giving nursing care, measures should be used which will help to prevent pain.

A. (1) Soft tissues should not be pinched or scraped.
   (2) Tubes should be inserted carefully.
   (3) Injured parts should be handled very carefully.
B. Injured parts should be kept well supported.
C. Changes of position should be made slowly and smoothly.
D. All tubes should be well lubricated before insertion.
E. Distention of tissue by too rapid a flow of fluid, or too much fluid, or high pressure of fluid should be avoided (e.g. in subcutaneous injections, enemas or tube feedings).
F. Drugs and solutions should be administered according to the route prescribed (e.g. intramuscularly or intravenously). (When there is infiltration of intravenous fluids, the flow of fluid into the tissues should be stopped.)
G. All equipment used in treatments should be checked for smoothness and good working order before use.
H. Any substances adhered to the skin or mucous membrane should be removed with proper solvents.
I. Caution should be observed in administering hot or cold applications.
J. Relaxation of voluntary muscles should be encouraged when they are involved in an examination or a treatment (e.g. gluteal muscle in intramuscular injection or perineal and sphincter muscles in enemas or catheterizations). (Emotional preparation for the procedure may be helpful.)
K. Pain-relieving drugs may be administered as ordered prior to treatments which may be painful.
L. Gradual increases in exercise should be encouraged.
M. When a patient has a nerve irritation, muscle spasm, or diminished arterial blood flow,
   (1) Muscular activity of the affected part should be limited.
   (2) Marked temperature changes of the affected part should be avoided.
N. Emotional support should be given prior to and/or during uncomfortable examinations or treatments.

4. Nursing measures which may be used to alleviate pain include:
   A. Alleviation of pressure.
      (1) A change in position may be helpful.
      (2) An injured part may be elevated.
      (3) Active or passive exercise may be used. (Exceptions include tender muscles or possible phlebothrombosis.)
      (4) Rectal tubes or enemas may be used as ordered.
      (5) Catheterization may be done as ordered.
      (6) Tight dressings or binders may be loosened unless contraindicated.
   B. Adjustment of position to provide for as near normal body alignment as possible.
   C. Application of heat or cold unless contraindicated.
   D. Reduction of any environmental factors which may be annoying to the patient (e.g. noise, light, odors or motion).
   E. Encouragement of relaxation of tense muscles which may be increasing discomfort (e.g. massage of tense neck muscles in tension headache).
   F. Emotional support.
   G. Administration of pain-relieving drugs as ordered.
      (1) Symptoms not yet evaluated by a physician should not be masked.
      (2) Any possible dependence upon drugs should be reported.
      (3) The time of administration of drugs should *prevent* severe pain.
5. When nausea is the physical discomfort, vomiting may be encouraged or discouraged as indicated. (See Nursing Care Related to "C.")
6. When hunger pangs occur, food and/or fluids should be provided within orders and as possible.
7. When a patient who is in a body cast feels uncomfortable upper abdominal fullness after eating, smaller meals may be given more frequently.
8. When thirst occurs,

A. Fluids should be provided within orders.
B. Oral hygiene or just moistening the mouth can be used if oral fluids are contraindicated or restricted.

9. When itching or a sensation of burning occurs,
   A. Cold wet compresses may be applied.
   B. A cooling lotion (e.g. witch hazel) may be applied unless contraindicated by such factors as open wounds or possible allergic response.
   C. Lanolin or cold cream may be applied to a dry skin.
   D. Calomine lotion may be applied to an unbroken skin.
   E. Antihistaminic drugs may be administered as ordered.
10. Tingling and numbness of an extremity should be reported promptly when:
    A. Improving circulation to the affected part fails to alleviate the symptoms.
       (1) Change of position may be helpful.
       (2) Massage may be used.
       (3) Constricting bandages may be loosened unless contraindicated.
    B. These symptoms occur frequently.
    C. These symptoms are associated with an applied cast or splint.
11. When a patient is unable to feel pain, special precautions should be taken to protect him from any type of physical injury.
12. When a patient is restless, unable to sleep, or unusually irritable and is either unaware of any physical discomfort or unable to communicate to others the cause of his discomfort, he should be observed thoroughly for the cause and appropriate actions should be taken. Possible causes include:
    A. Bleeding. (See Nursing Care Related to "A.")
    B. Poor peripheral circulation. (See Nursing Care Related to "A.")
    C. Irritation of the skin or mucous membrane. (See Nursing Care Related to "L.")
    D. Infiltration of intravenous fluids. (See Nursing Care Related to "N.")
    E. Poor body alignment. (See Nursing Care Related to "K.")

F. Distention of the gastro-intestinal tract. (See Nursing Care Related to "I.")
G. Urinary retention. (See Nursing Care Related to "D.")
H. Thirst. (See Nursing Care Related to "D.")
I. Hunger. (See Nursing Care Related to "C.")

PRINCIPLES OF ANATOMY AND PHYSIOLOGY UNDERLYING THE NURSING CARE

N. Sensations of physical discomfort may indicate injury or threat of injury to the body.

1. The simplest and most widely distributed sensation is that of pain.
   A. Several kinds of stimuli are adequate to elicit pain (e.g. electrical, mechanical, chemical and thermal).
      (1) Pressure against pain fibers causes pain.
      (2) Continued pressure against a nerve can result in tingling sensations and numbness.
      (3) Strong stimulation of sensory receptors for heat or cold may cause pain.
      (4) Chemicals which injure tissues (e.g. strong acids) cause pain.
   B. Some regions of the body give rise primarily, or almost exclusively, to the sensation of pain (e.g. the teeth, tympanic membrane or cornea).
      (Localization of pain is difficult when an area is supplied primarily by pain fibers.)
   C. Muscles and tendons possess exquisite pain sensitivity.
      (1) Exercising ischemic muscles usually results in severe cramping pain.
      (2) Lameness may result from exercising muscles which have been used relatively little for a prolonged period of time.
      (3) Muscles are very sensitive to pinching or squeezing.
   D. Pain fibers adapt very slowly, if at all.
   E. Prolonged cold decreases the sensitivity of sensory receptors.
   F. Mucous membrane has fewer sensory receptors for pain than does the skin.

2. The 3 kinds of pain which are generally recognized and designated are:
   A. Superficial or cutaneous.
   B. Deep (from muscles, tendons, joints and fascia).
   C. Visceral.
3. The viscera are relatively insensitive to ordinary types of stimuli, but pain may result from:
   A. Tension or stretch of smooth muscle fibers.
   B. Chemical irritation, especially when the organ is ischemic (e.g. myocardial infraction or strangulated hernia).
4. Irritation of the viscera may be manifested by:
   A. Referred pain.
      (1) Pain is felt in the body surface though originating in the viscera.
      (2) Pain is felt in dermatomes associated (because of their nerve supplies) with posterior roots through which the afferent impulses from the viscera reach the spinal cord (e.g. heart pain may be felt in upper shoulders and possibly radiating down the arms).
   B. Poorly localized pain.
   C. Excessive sensitivity to pain and pressure over and around affected organ.
   D. Autonomic reflexes (e.g. sweating or vasomotor changes).
   E. Somatic reflexes (e.g. muscular rigidity over the affected area).
5. A painful stimulus (visceral) is received by a visceral receptor and impulses are transmitted to the brain by the following routes:
   A. To the spinal cord and to the thalamus via the spino-thalamic tract.
   B. Directly to the thalamus via a cranial nerve. (Irritation of the trigeminal nerve may cause pain in all the areas supplied by the trigeminal nerve (e.g. face and buccal cavity).)
6. A painful stimulus (cutaneous or deep) is received by a somatic receptor carried to the spinal cord by a spinal nerve, across the gray commissure, and to the spino-thalamic tract to the thalamus.

7. The thalamus gives rise to a crude, uncritical form of consciousness, and diffuse and unlocalized pain may be perceived at this level.
8. Sensory fibers for pain pass from the thalamus to the somesthetic area of the cerebral cortex where more discriminative perception of pain may be made.
9. If the axon of a specific nerve fiber or its dorsal root is irritated, pain is perceived as coming from the terminal end.
10. The brain tissue itself has no pain receptors, but pain in the head may result from:
    - A. Stimulation of receptors in the intra-cranial blood vessels which may be due to changes in intracranial pressure or to local vasodilatation.
    - B. Increased tension of posterior neck muscles (e.g. due to emotional tension or meningeal irritation).
    - C. Constipation (reflex in nature).
11. Pain may be felt as sharp, stabbing, burning, cramping, throbbing, dull, aching, or as a sensation of tenderness.
12. The perception threshold of pain remains remarkably constant among normal persons but may be altered by various influences which may include:
    - A. Pressure against painful area.
    - B. Warmth applied to painful area.
    - C. Hypnosis.
    - D. Drugs (e.g. analgesics, narcotics).
13. Individual reactions to pain may include:
    - A. Contractions of facial muscles.
    - B. Vocalization.
    - C. Vasomotor responses.
        - (1) Skin color changes.
        - (2) Pulse and blood pressure changes.
    - D. Sweating.
    - E. Respiratory changes (e.g. hyperventilation).
    - F. Increased muscular tension (local and/or generalized).
    - G. Nausea and vomiting.
14. An individual's threshold of reaction to pain varies with learning and temperament.

15. The thalamus plays an important role in the affects of various sensations. (Pain has an unpleasant affect.)
16. The hypothalamus is closely related to both autonomic responses and to the prefrontal lobe of the cerebrum. (Prefrontal lobe activity is closely associated with an individual's emotional reactions.)
17. Uncomfortable organic sensations (other than pain) include hunger, thirst, nausea, itching or tickling, feelings of fullness in the viscera (e.g. stomach, rectum or bladder).
    A. Hunger pangs result from the contractions of the muscular wall of an empty stomach.
    B. Nausea usually precedes vomiting but may occur without it.
        (1) Nausea may be accompanied by sweating.
        (2) Nausea may be accompanied by excessive salivation.
    C. Thirst may result from either dryness of the pharyngeal mucosa or general cellular dehydration.
    D. Irritation of sensory receptors of the bladder or urethra may result in a strong desire to void and frequency in urination.
    E. The cause of itching or tickling is unknown but it is closely associated with such factors as:
        (1) Dryness of the skin.
        (2) Some skin lesions (e.g. in measles or chicken pox).
        (3) Urticaria.
        (4) Jaundice.
        (5) Emotional disturbances.
18. Unpleasant organic sensations may cause:
    A. Restlessness and bad dreams.
    B. Sleeplessness.
    C. Emotional tension (e.g. with symptoms of anxiety).
    D. Increased irritability to stimuli.

PRINCIPLES OF PHYSICS UNDERLYING THE NURSING CARE

N. Sensations of physical discomfort may indicate injury or threat of injury to the body.

1. Friction is that force which opposes motion between 2 contacting surfaces.
   A. Friction is caused by surface irregularities.
   B. Friction may be decreased by decreasing the irregularities (e.g. through smoothing the surfaces or separating the surfaces with lubrication).
2. Pressure is the force exerted on a unit area. (Fluids flow from an area of higher pressure to one of lower pressure, and the rate of volume flow is directly related to the pressure gradient.)

Section O: Nursing Care and Science Principles Related to Vision, Hearing, Smell, Taste, Touch and the Discernment of Temperature.

O. Vision, hearing, smell, taste, touch and discernment of temperature afford the body with information about the external environment.

NURSING CARE

1. Patients should be observed for signs and symptoms of visual disturbances and injuries to the eye, and these should be reported. This is of particular importance when the patient:
   A. Is an infant or young child.
   B. Is aged.
   C. Has a congenital condition, surgical condition, disease condition or injury which involves—or may involve:
      (1) The eyeball.
      (2) The eyelid.
      (3) The extrinsic eye muscles.
      (4) Nervous tissue concerned with vision.
2. Reportable signs and symptoms of abnormal conditions of those body parts concerned with vision may include:
   A. Visual disturbances (e.g. partial or total blindness, blurring of vision, spots before the eyes, diplopia, light halos or visual hallucinations).
   B. Abnormal positions or movements of the eyeballs.
   C. Abnormal changes in pupil size (e.g. irregularity, prolonged dilation or constriction).
   D. Difficulties in postural adjustments, handling of objects and so forth.

E. Photophobia.
F. Pain (e.g. frontal, occipital or in or behind eyes).
G. Frowning, squinting, muscular twitching in eyelids or around the eyes.
H. Excessive blinking, redness or burning of the conjunctiva.
I. Edema of the eyelid, itching of the eyelids.
J. Abnormal drainage from the eye (e.g. pus or excessive tears).
K. Bleeding in, from or around the eyeball.
L. Vertigo.
M. Nausea and vomiting.
N. Inability to open or close the eye.

3. Patients should be protected from injury to the eye by such methods as:
   A. Providing appropriate lighting. (When pupils are dilated, bright lights should be avoided.)
   B. Using caution when manipulating objects close to the eye.
   C. Protecting the eyes from foreign objects or friction.
   D. Protecting the eyes from any injurious chemicals or physical agents.
   E. Providing appropriate therapeutic care promptly when there is injury to the eye.
4. When a patient has injury to the eye, the affected eye may be temporarily covered prior to medical examination. (Injured eyes should be protected from bright lights.)
5. When a patient has facial paralysis involving the orbicularis muscle, is unconscious or has corneal anesthesia, the eye(s) should be protected by such methods as:
   A. Temporary covering.
   B. Frequent moistening and cleansing of the conjunctiva.
6. When the eye is moistened and/or cleansed, physiological saline solution should be used. (In case of emergency, water may be used.)
7. When a patient has surgery involving the eyeball (e.g. cataract removal),
   A. The physician's orders concerning the following should be carried out *specifically*:
      (1) The use of protective covering over the eyes.

(2) Lighting.
(3) Positioning.
(4) The amount of physical activity.
(5) The diet.
(6) Bowel elimination.

B. Stability of the head should be promoted.
C. Sneezing, coughing and stooping should be discouraged.

8. When a patient has increased intra-ocular pressure,
   A. Factors causing sudden marked changes in blood pressure should be avoided.
   B. Using the eyes in a dim light may be discouraged.
9. When a patient is partially or totally blind,
   A. He should be given adequate information about his environment.
   B. His immediate environment should be arranged in such a way as to help him in meeting his needs satisfactorily.
10. When an artificial eye is used, provision should be made for cleansing of the eye socket.
11. All patients should be observed for signs and symptoms of auditory disturbances and ear injuries and these should be reported. This is of particular importance when the patient:
    A. Is an infant or a young child.
    B. Is aged.
    C. Has a congenital condition, surgical condition, disease condition or injury which involves—or may involve—either the ear or nervous tissue involved with hearing.
    D. Is receiving drugs which may cause auditory disturbances.
12. Reportable signs and symptoms of abnormal conditions of those body parts concerned with hearing may include:
    A. Auditory disturbances (e.g. deafness, tinnitus or auditory hallucinations).
    B. Nystagmus.
    C. Dizziness.
    D. Nausea and vomiting.
    E. Pain (e.g. headache, pain in ear or in mastoid region).
    F. Feeling of fullness in ears.
    G. Abnormal discharge from the ear.
    H. Swelling behind the ear.

13. Ear injuries should be prevented by such methods as:
    A. Protecting the auditory canal from foreign objects.
    B. Preventing friction against or distortion of the pinna.
    C. Discouraging blowing of the nose.
    D. Discouraging the bottle-feeding of infants when they are lying flat on their backs.
    E. Providing appropriate therapeutic care promptly when there is question of ear injury or nose or throat infection.
14. When a patient has injury to the ear (including surgery),
    A. The physician's orders concerning the following should be carried out *specifically*:
       (1) The use of protective covering over the ear.
       (2) Positioning.
       (3) The amount of physical activity.
       (4) The diet.
    B. Stability of the head should be promoted.
    C. Mechanical injury to the ear should be avoided during treatments involving the ear.
    D. Aseptic technics should be observed in the care of the ear and this is of particular importance when there is an opening into the middle or inner ear.
    E. Nose-blowing should be discouraged.
15. When a patient has surgery or an infection involving the middle ear, he should be observed closely for signs and symptoms of injury to the facial nerve. These signs and symptoms include:
    A. Inability to close eye on affected side.
    B. Inability to use facial expression on affected side.
    C. The mouth drawn over to the unaffected side.
16. When a patient's auditory canal has become plugged with cerumen or a foreign object, he should be discouraged from cleaning it himself and encouraged to seek the aid of a physician. (The affected ear should be examined prior to any irrigations.)
17. When any solution is administered into the auditory canal, the solution should be at body temperature.
18. When atmospheric pressure changes cause pressure against

the tympanic membrane, discomfort may be relieved by:
 A. Frequent swallowing.
 B. Yawning.

19. Patients should be protected from noise.
20. When a patient is partially or totally deaf, he should be afforded means of communication which will serve satisfactorily in helping him to meet his needs.
21. Appropriate verbal communications should be used when caring for a comatose patient.
22. Patients should be observed for their abilities to perceive superficial touch and pressure and abnormalities should be reported. This is of particular importance when there is injury, or possible injury, to peripheral nerves, the spinal cord and/or the brain.
23. When a patient is unable to perceive superficial pressure and/or touch, he may need assistance with some locomotor activities.
24. Patients should be observed for their abilities to perceive taste and smell and abnormalities should be reported. This is of particular importance when there is injury, or possible injury, to the brain.
25. When the senses of taste and/or smell are diminished (e.g. during upper respiratory infections or in old age), high flavoring of food may be helpful in encouraging eating.
26. When a bitter-tasting drug is administered orally,
    A. The dissolving of a solid medication in the mouth may be discouraged.
    B. The tongue may be avoided during the swallowing of a liquid medication (e.g. with use of drinking tube).
    C. The mouth may be rinsed well after administration of the drug.

PRINCIPLES OF ANATOMY AND PHYSIOLOGY UNDERLYING THE NURSING CARE

O. Vision, hearing, smell, taste, touch and discernment of temperature afford the body with information about the external environment.

Facts Related to Vision

1. The eye, the organ of vision, is a spherical body lying within a bony orbit.
2. The wall of the eyeball consists of 3 concentric layers.
   A. The external layer consists of:
      (1) The sclera, a white fibrous covering of the sides and posterior part.
      (2) The cornea, a transparent tissue of the anterior region.
   B. The middle layer consists of:
      (1) The choroid, containing many blood vessels.
      (2) The ciliary body.
      (3) The iris, a muscular diaphragm which has a circular aperture called the pupil.
   C. The innermost coat, the retina, which lines the posterior part and sides of the eyeball and contains the receptors for the optic nerve.
3. The cavity of the eye contains:
   A. The aqueous humor, a watery fluid which fills the space between the cornea and the lens.
   B. The vitreous body, a gelatinous substance which fills the cavity posterior to the lens.
   C. The crystalline lens, a transparent, biconvex circular structure which lies behind the center of the pupil.
4. The exposed part of the eyeball is covered by delicate epithelial tissue, the conjunctiva, which is reflected onto the inner surfaces of the eyelids.
5. The conjunctival surfaces are kept moist and clean by a film of tears, a slightly hypertonic, clear and watery fluid, secreted by the lacrimal glands.
   A. Tears are delivered through several fine ducts into the conjunctival fornix.
   B. Continuous reflex movements of the eyelids keep the exposed cornea moist with tears.
   C. Tears drain through the lacrimal duct to the nose. (This process is dependent upon blinking and gravity.)
   D. Tear secretion is induced reflexly by stimulation of the

cornea or conjunctiva. (This reflex may be annulled by either interference with the sensory nerves from the cornea or conjunctiva or with the motor nerves supplying the lacrimal gland.)

E. Fluids having a salt concentration greater than 1.5 per cent or less than 0.16 per cent are irritating to the eyes of most people.

6. The cornea is supplied by a rich plexus of pain fibers which have a low threshold.
7. The eyeball has a relatively large blood supply to the choroid, to the internal surface of the eyeball and to the conjunctiva. (Capillary hemorrhage in the internal surface of the eye, such as may occur when there is peripheral vascular disease, causes visual disturbances.)
8. The intra-ocular fluids are produced continually and drain through tiny channels into some of the veins of the eye.
   - A. The normal intra-ocular pressure of fluids in the eye chambers is 20 to 25 mm. of mercury.
   - B. The intra-ocular pressure reflects very closely changes in the choroidal capillary and venous blood pressures (e.g. a rise or fall in the arterial blood pressure may cause a corresponding change in the intra-ocular pressure).
   - C. Dark adaptation causes increased intra-ocular pressure.
   - D. Increased ocular pressure causes compression of the blood vessels of the eye and subsequent interference with the total eyeball.
9. The optic nerve, formed by many nerve fibers from the retina, leaves the eyeball at a point called the optic disc.
10. The optic nerves pass backwards to the optic chiasm where some fibers cross to the opposite side. From here the two optic tracts pass backwards through the midbrain and, eventually, to the visual cortex in the occipital lobe of the cerebrum.
    - A. Areas in the midbrain contain centers which serve to correlate eye movements and movements of the eyelids and body which protect the eye from injury.
    - B. Sensations of light are perceived in the visual cortex.
    - C. Interference with any part of the optic nerves, chiasm or

tracts, by such means as pressure, causes visual defects.

D. "Conscious vision" probably is a function of large portions of the cerebral cortex.

11. Blinking, a voluntary or reflex act, is accomplished by movements of the eyelids.
    A. Movement of the eyelids helps to protect the eye from the entrance of foreign particles.
    B. Closure of the eyes is accomplished by the contraction of muscles around the eye which are under the control of branches of the facial nerve.
    C. Opening of the eyes is accomplished by the contraction of muscles of the eyelid under the control of the oculomotor nerve.
    D. Stimulation of the cornea or conjunctiva normally causes blinking.
12. Light rays enter the eye through the pupil and their refraction, primarily through the cornea and crystalline lens, normally cause them to focus on the retina.
    A. The iris serves as an opaque screen which adjusts the amount of light allowed to enter the eye.
        (1) Parasympathetic stimulation of circular muscles in the iris cause constriction of the pupil.
        (2) Sympathetic stimulation of radial muscles in the iris cause dilation of the pupil.
        (3) In bright illumination the pupil is constricted, while in dim illumination the pupil is dilated.
        (4) Constriction of the pupil helps to prevent blurred images.
    B. The adjustment of the eye whereby it is able to focus the image of both near and far objects on the retina is called accommodation.
        (1) Accommodation is accomplished by changes in the convexity of the anterior surface of the crystalline lens.
        (2) Convergence of the eyes and constriction of the pupils occur when there is accommodation for near objects.

(3) The accommodation reaction originates in the visual cortex.

(4) Generally, the ability to accommodate is fairly poor in a child up to the age of 2 to 3 years.

(5) Generally, the ability to accommodate decreases after the age of 45.

C. If the image is focused in front of or behind the retina, vision is abnormal.

D. Chemical changes occurring in the lens may cause it to become opaque.

E. Abnormal curvatures of the cornea result in astigmatism.

F. Abnormalities in vision due to faulty accommodation or an abnormally curved cornea may be corrected by specially ground lenses placed in front of the cornea.

13. The retina is stimulated most effectively by light but crude visual sensations can be evoked by mechanical forms of stimulation (e.g. pressure).

14. Concentrated sources of light situated near an object being observed causes glare.

A. When there is glare, visual acuity is decreased and eye strain occurs.

B. Squinting helps to reduce glare.

15. The constant use of the eyes in poor lighting leads to ocular strain and fatigue.

16. How much illumination is desirable for ideal vision depends largely upon such factors as the amount of visual acuity demanded for the job and the contrast between light and dark in what is being observed. (A general over-all illumination of a room with an increased illumination on the working surface produces a minimum of eyestrain and glare.)

17. The extrinsic eye muscles move the eyeball in its orbit.

A. The eye muscle movements are under the control of cranial nerves. (Voluntary movements are controlled by the motor cortex.)

B. At birth the eyes are not associated with each other but act as 2 independent sense organs. By about the third month the child begins, by trial and error process, to move his eyeballs in such a way as to gain a common visual direction and, in this way, his eyes can become associated.

C. Diplopia can occur because of weakness of muscles in one eye or imbalance between muscles of both eyes.

D. Eye and head movements are closely associated with the vestibular apparatus.

(1) Nystagmus involves eye movements caused by the stimulation of eye muscle nerves through the vestibular nuclei.

(2) Visual disturbances are often associated with vertigo and nausea.

18. Binocular vision is important for depth perception and for the largest possible visual field.

19. Photophobia due to excessive light is probably due to referred pain.

Facts Related to Hearing

1. The ear is the organ of hearing and is composed of 3 parts.

A. The external auditory canal is an S-shaped passage approximately 1¼ inches long which ends blindly at the flexible tympanic membrane. It is lined with skin which contains cerumen-secreting glands. (The ear canal in a child is relatively straight but changes occur in the direction of the canal during growth.)

B. The middle ear is a tiny chamber situated in the temporal bone containing three articulating miniature bones: the malleus articulates with the tympanic membrane, the incus is in the center and the stapes articulates with the oval window in the posterior wall.

(1) The middle ear is filled with air maintained at atmospheric pressure by means of an air passageway through the Eustachian tube.

(2) The middle ear is lined with mucous membrane which is continuous with that of the Eustachian tube and nasopharynx and the mastoid antrum.

C. The internal ear, also in the temporal bone, contains the semicircular canals and the cochlea.

(1) The cochlea and semicircular canals contain 2 fluids, separated by membrane. (One of the fluids is cerebrospinal fluid which reaches the cochlea through a duct from the subarachnoid space.)

(2) The cochlea contains the auditory sense receptors which transmit impulses to the auditory nerve.

(3) The semicircular canals are concerned with equilibrium. (The fluid in the semicircular canals, when heated or cooled quickly, gives rise to sensations of position change which may result in vertigo.)

2. The cochlear division of the auditory nerve leaves the cochlea, passes to the midbrain (here there are centers for auditory reflexes) and, then, passes to the temporal lobe of the cerebral cortex for conscious perception. (Hearing is generally the last sense to be lost when there is loss of consciousness.)
3. Normally, the tympanic membrane is forced into vibrations by sound waves and the vibratory motions are transmitted through the ossicles to the fluid in the inner ear. (Any interference with the transmission of vibrations or with the nervous tissue concerned with the sense of hearing will result in some degree of deafness. In old age, movement of the ossicles may be decreased.)
4. The posterior wall of the middle ear has an opening into the mastoid antrum.
   A. The mastoid contains a deep groove for the lateral sinus of the brain.
   B. The mastoid antrum is separated from the brain by only a thin plate of bone.
5. A branch of the facial nerve lies very close to the middle ear. (If the trunk of the facial nerve is injured, all the muscles of the affected side of the face are paralyzed.)
6. Continued stimulation of the auditory nerves gives rise to general fatigue and nervous irritability.
7. The pinna of the external ear contains elastic cartilage and is covered with skin.

Facts Related to Superficial Touch and Pressure

1. Objects brought into contact with the skin produce the sensation of touch or pressure through the stimulation of end organs located in the skin and subcutaneous tissues.
2. Nerve fibers which carry impulses of touch and pressure from the periphery to the brain either pass:
   A. Up the cord in the posterior columns (gracilis and cuneatus tracts) and cross in the medulla, or
   B. Up the anterolateral spinothalamic tracts, crossing at different levels of the cord.
3. Sensations of pressure and touch are perceived in the somatic sensory area of the cerebral cortex, primarily in the postcentral gyrus.

Facts Related to Taste and Smell

1. The olfactory end organs are located in the nasal mucosa.
2. The sensation of smell is perceived in the temporal lobe of the cerebral cortex.
3. The taste buds are embedded in the tongue and are sensitive to substances in solution. (The number of functioning taste buds decreases with age.)

Facts Related to Discernment of Heat and Cold

1. The receptors for heat and cold are located in skin and mucous membranes. (Mucous membrane has fewer sensory nerve endings for heat and cold than has the skin.)
2. Sensory impulses for heat and cold travel through peripheral nerves to the spinal cord, up the spinal cord via the lateral spino-thalamic tracts, through the medulla, to the thalamus and, finally to the cerebral cortex where the sensation is interpreted.

PRINCIPLES OF PHYSICS UNDERLYING THE NURSING CARE

O. Vision, hearing, smell, taste, touch and discernment of temperature afford the body with information about the external environment.

1. Light is a form of electromagnetic radiation (gamma rays, x-rays, ultra-violet rays, visible light rays and infra-red rays).
2. Illumination varies with 3 factors:
   A. The power of the source of light.
   B. The distance from the source of light.
   C. The angle of incidence at which the light strikes a surface and is reflected.
3. Refraction is the bending of a ray of light when it passes from one medium to another of a different density.
4. A coverging lens causes, through refraction, the convergence of parallel light rays on the opposite side of the lens at a point called the principal focus.
5. Sound, which is within limits of hearing in human beings, originates in vibrations within a definite frequency range; and the waves which are set up travel outward from the source in some medium (solid, liquid or gas).
6. Pressure is the force exerted on a unit area.
7. Pressure exerted on a confined liquid is transmitted undiminished to all parts of that liquid.
8. Gravitation is the force of attraction between 2 objects (e.g. the earth and an object on or near the earth).

PRINCIPLES OF CHEMISTRY UNDERLYING THE NURSING CARE

O. Vision, hearing, smell, taste, touch and discernment of temperature afford the body with information about the external environment.

1. An isotonic solution is one which exerts the same osmotic pressure as a solution on the other side of a semi-permeable membrane. A physiological saline solution (isotonic with body fluids) is approximately a 0.9 per cent aqueous solution of sodium chloride.

Section P: Nursing Care and Science Principles Related to Cognition and the Association of Ideas.

P. Normal functioning of the cerebral cortex is essential to the mental faculties of cognition and association of ideas.

NURSING CARE

1. All patients should be observed for signs and symptoms of impairment of their mental faculties, and these should be reported. This is of particular importance when there is:
   A. Brain pathology or head injury (possible or actual).
   B. Impairment of general circulation or local circulation to the brain.
   C. Anoxia.
   D. Fever.
   E. Infectious disease (e.g. encephalitis, measles or mumps).
   F. Toxic substances in the blood stream (e.g. anesthetics or barbituates).
   G. Emotional disturbance.
2. Reportable signs and symptoms of the impairment of mental faculties may include:
   A. Inability to remember (recent or remote).
   B. Faulty sensory perceptions, confusion.
   C. Inability to reason.
   D. Changes in the usual behavior patterns.
3. When a patient shows signs of impairment of his mental faculties,
   A. He should be carefully protected from harming himself

or others (e.g. close observation and controlling environment).

B. He should be helped as much as necessary or possible in meeting his basic physiological needs.

PRINCIPLES OF ANATOMY AND PHYSIOLOGY UNDERLYING THE NURSING CARE

P. Normal functioning of the cerebral cortex is essential to the mental faculties of cognition and association of ideas.

1. The cortical gray matter is the chief organ of the psychic life of man.
2. The mental capacity of an individual seems to be a function of the cerebral cortex as a whole (e.g. the quantity of cortex may be more important than any actual location).
3. The association areas of the cerebral cortex (located in all lobes) are those areas in which complex sensory, motor and behavior patterns are integrated. (Extensive association areas seem to be located in the temporal lobes.)
4. Perception is a function of the cerebral cortex. (Perception implies the dynamic organization of external and internal stimuli into a meaningful whole and this organization is one of the determinants of behavior.)
5. Gradual development of the mental faculties occurs during the normal growth and development of individuals.

Section Q: Nursing Care and Science Principles Related to Speech.

Q. Speech provides one means of communication.

NURSING CARE

1. All patients should be observed for signs and symptoms of their inability to use speech effectively, and abnormalities should be reported. This is of particular importance when:
   A. The patient is a child.
   B. There is a possibility of or actual brain damage.
   C. There is a condition involving the anatomical structures concerned with the production of sound and the formation of words.
   D. There is a possibility of deafness.
2. Reportable signs and symptoms of problems with speech may include:
   A. Inability to make sounds.
   B. Hoarseness.
   C. Production of words and/or sounds which cannot be understood.
   D. Inappropriate speech.
   E. Confused speech.
   F. Inability to express self in spoken and/or written word.
   G. Inappropriate response to the spoken and/or written word.
3. When a patient is unable to use his voice for communication, it is necessary to use writing or some other means of communication.
4. When a patient is unable to use or to understand speech

effectively, it is necessary to observe him closely for other methods of communication and to develop different methods for communication.

PRINCIPLES OF ANATOMY AND PHYSIOLOGY UNDERLYING THE NURSING CARE

Q. Speech provides one means of communication.

1. The larynx produces vocal sounds, but the actual articulation of words is accomplished by the shape given to the mouth and throat and the movement and positions of the lips and tongue.
   A. Vocal sounds are produced by the vibration of the vocal folds in the larynx caused by the controlled passage of air through the larynx.
   B. The length and tension of the vocal cords determine the pitch of the voice. (Changes in the position and tension of the vocal folds are brought about largely by intrinsic muscles which move some of the cartilages of the larynx.)
2. The function of speech involves both sensory and motor elements in the use and understanding of symbols for the expression of ideas.
   A. The function of speech includes, on the sensory side, the abilities to understand both the written and the spoken word.
   B. The function of speech includes, on the motor side, the abilities both to speak and to write words.
3. The function of speech is thought to involve the cerebral cortex as a whole.
   A. The motor speech area (Broca's area) is located in the motor area of the frontal lobe of the cerebral hemisphere which is not dominant (e.g. left hemisphere in a right-handed person).
   B. The sensory areas of speech are considered to be largely in the occipital and temporal lobes.
4. Speech is learned.
   A. Speaking is learned by imitation and generally the for-

mulation of intelligible words by a child begins at 9 to 18 months of life.

B. Understanding the spoken word starts early in life, generally in a few months.

C. Writing and understanding the written word can be learned generally after the fourth or fifth year.

Nursing Care and Science Principles Related to the Prevention of Microbial Injury

NURSING CARE

1. The immediate environment (e.g. furniture, bedding, clothing, walls and floor) should be free from dust, dirt and organic material such as food or body discharges.
2. Air currents should be controlled and good ventilation promoted.
3. Objects which may harbor micro-organisms may be exposed to direct sunlight for extended periods of time.
4. Insects should be controlled.
5. The skin, hair, nails and exposed mucous membranes should be clean.
   A. The skin should be free from excessive moisture.
   B. Frequent, thorough handwashing should be promoted. (This is particularly important prior to eating or preparing foods.)
   C. Special hand and arm cleansing (e.g. scrubbing) should be employed by personnel prior to performing sterile procedures and following contamination by infective, or potentially infective, material.
   D. Special cleansing technics should be applied in the care of the skin and mucous membrane of the patient prior to:
      (1) Surgical incisions.
      (2) Injections.
      (3) The introduction of a tube into the urethra.
   E. The nipples should be clean before nursing an infant.
   F. All wounds should be thoroughly cleansed and should be covered as indicated by need for cleanliness.

G. The skin or mucous membrane around open wounds should be kept clean.

H. Open wounds should be protected from possible contaminants (e.g. hair, dust, lint, respiratory secretions or fecal material).

I. The destruction of normal flora of mucous membranes by frequent irrigations or over-use of antiseptic solutions should be discouraged.

6. All utensils which are put in or around the mouth should be clean.
7. Fingers should be kept away from the nose and mouth.
8. All equipment used in nursing care should be free from dust, dirt and organic material such as body discharges.
9. Only disinfected and/or sterile equipment should be used in contact with or close to broken skin or mucous membrane or in parts of the body which are normally free from microbial growth.
10. Effective technics for disinfection and sterilization should be employed.
11. Respiratory secretions, saliva, feces, urine, blood and exudates should be handled as potentially infective and proper disposal of them should be made. (Vomitus and vaginal secretions may be considered to be potentially infective.)
12. Technics for the isolation of patients should be carried out as ordered by the physician and/or indicated by the diagnosis of the patient.

A. Isolation requirements will vary depending upon:

(1) Where the organisms are in the host and what the portal of exit is.

(2) The modes of transmission of the organisms.

(3) The portal of entry for the organisms.

(4) The nature of the organism.

B. All materials in direct or indirect contact with a patient who has an infection which can be transmitted to others or can re-infect him (through respiratory secretions, saliva, urine, vomitus, feces or exudates) must be considered to be contaminated with pathogenic microorganisms.

(1) All articles of furniture, walls, floors and so forth in the area of the patient should be kept in a clean condition at all times, and meticulous cleaning should be done upon discharge of the patient.

(2) Fomites should be burned after use or, if the contaminated article is to be used again, it should be disinfected or sterilized. (Either should be done as soon as possible.)

C. Infective body discharges (e.g. feces or sputum) should be disinfected and/or disposed of safely.

D. Gowns or change of clothing may be used to protect clothing from infective materials.

E. Face masks may be worn either to prevent contamination by respiratory secretions or to prevent inhalation of pathogenic organisms from the air.

(1) When used to prevent the inhalation of pathogenic organisms from the air, face masks should be changed at least every hour and oftener if moist.

(2) Other means of controlling the spread of respiratory secretions include the proper use of disposable tissues and the control of coughing or sneezing.

F. Gloves may be worn to protect the skin of the hands from infective material.

G. Special goggles can be used to protect the eyes from infective material.

13. Individuals with the following symptoms should be suspected of possible infection, and precautions relative to the protection of self and others from the infection should be employed:

A. Fever.

B. Lesions of skin and mucous membranes.

C. Discomfort in normal body processes (e.g. painful swallowing or burning upon voiding).

E. Vomiting and/or diarrhea.

F. Abnormal drainage (e.g. pus).

14. Immunizations for smallpox, pertussis, tetanus, diphtheria and poliomyelitis should be encouraged for infants and young children.

A. Immunizations against typhoid fever may be encouraged in some localities.

B. Immunizations against these and other diseases may be encouraged for children and adults as indicated by the possibility of infection.

15. When children up to the age of 2 years, at least, have been exposed to the measles, their parents should be encouraged to talk with their physicians about the exposure.
16. Women should be encouraged to seek obstetrical care early in their pregnancies.
17. All food, milk, water and ice should be kept clean.
    A. Raw milk (unless certified) should not be used.
    B. The use of unpasteurized milk products should be discouraged.
    C. The preparation of food or food handling by persons who have infections which may be transmitted by respiratory secretions, feces, urine, saliva or exudates should be discouraged.
18. Milk should be kept properly refrigerated at all times.
19. Foods which spoil easily or often act as excellent culture media for micro-organisms (e.g. prepared cream dishes or chopped meats) should be kept properly refrigerated.
20. Meat and fish should be thoroughly cooked.
21. Any canned foods (especially home-canned foods) which have a bad odor and the liquid of which contains bubbles of gas should not be eaten.

PRINCIPLES OF MICROBIOLOGY UNDERLYING THE NURSING CARE

Facts Pertaining to Micro-organisms in General

1. There are many varieties of micro-organisms; most are harmless; few are pathogenic.
2. Some disease conditions in man are caused by micro-organisms.
   A. Micro-organisms cause all the diseases which can be spread from person to person (i.e. communicable diseases).

B. Infections are caused by disease-producing micro-organisms.
   (1) True pathogens are virulent organisms which possess invasive ability.
   (2) Some micro-organisms are not truly pathogenic but when given the opportunity they are able to cause disease.

C. The protozoa are microscopic animals and some varieties can cause disease in man.

D. Important microscopic plants which cause disease in man include the yeasts, molds and bacteria.
   (1) The basic morphological forms of simple bacteria are cocci, bacilli and spirilli.
   (2) The higher bacteria include the moldlike bacteria (e.g. mycobacteria).
   (3) Bacteria are capable of an extremely rapid rate of reproduction. (Cell division may take place as rapidly as every 20 minutes.)

E. Important ultra-microscopic forms of life which cause disease in man include the rickettsia and viruses.

4. Some bacteria give rise to resistant forms know as spores.
5. Some bacterial and protozoan forms possess flagella and can move in fluid, but other micro-organisms are not able to move themselves.

Facts Pertaining to the Control of Micro-organisms

1. Most pathogenic micro-organisms are mesophilic.
   A. Micro-organisms are not readily killed by low temperatures but may be prevented from active growth by low temperatures. (Freezing of water does not necessarily destroy the microbial content.)
   B. Most pathogenic micro-organisms can be killed at a temperature above 60° C. (140° F.), but mature spores may survive many hours of boiling temperature.
   C. All living organisms can be killed by exposure to moist heat at a temperature of 121° C. (250° F.) for 15 minutes.
2. All micro-organisms need moisture for growth. (Drying in-

hibits microbial growth but is an unreliable way of killing micro-organisms.)

3. All pathogenic micro-organisms require organic food. (Cleanliness—freedom from dirt and organic materials such as body discharges and foods—discourages the growth of micro-organisms.)
4. Direct ultra-violet rays will kill many types of pathogenic micro-organisms if there is ample exposure.
5. Chemicals which interfere with the life processes of micro-organisms will kill them or inhibit their growth and reproduction.
6. Sterilization is a process whereby all micro-organisms are destroyed. (Sterilization may be accomplished by incineration, autoclaving, prolonged boiling and dry heat.)
7. Disinfection is a process whereby most susceptible pathogenic non-sporing forms of micro-organisms are destroyed.
   A. Disinfection may be accomplished by boiling or chemicals (except spores).
   B. Raw milk can be disinfected by pasteurization.
   C. Water can be disinfected by proper chlorination.
8. Bacteriostasis is a process whereby the growth and reproduction of micro-organisms are prevented. (Bacteriostasis may be accomplished by cold, drying and chemicals.)
9. The effectiveness of various methods of disinfection and sterilization is dependent upon:
   A. The concentration of the chemical or the intensity of the physical agent used.
   B. The time allowed for the process.
   C. The nature of the material being treated. (The presence of organic material on objects interferes with disinfection and sterilization.)
   D. The type of organisms to be destroyed.
   E. The numbers of micro-organisms present.

Facts Pertaining to the Sources of Disease-Producing Micro-organisms

1. The major source of infection for communicable diseases is some person or animal who is discharging living pathogenic

organisms. (Carriers are persons who do not actually have clinical manifestations of an infection but may be sources of pathogenic organisms.)

2. Some bacteria normally present on or in the body may become opportunists and cause an infection.
   A. Micro-organisms are always present on the outer surfaces of the body and in cavities and tubes which have direct connection with outside of the body.
      (1) Persistently present on the skin are streptococci, staphylococci and some diphtheroids.
      (2) The mouth and throat receive many types of micro-organisms (e.g. lactobacilli).
      (3) The nasal passages are constantly contaminated by inhaled air but do not normally favor the growth of any organisms.
      (4) The external genitalia has normal flora and usually (especially in the female) has some fecal organisms.
      (5) The vagina has many organisms, normally, including lactobacilli.
   B. Micro-organisms do not regularly colonize in the stomach, bladder, uterus, trachea or lungs so these organs are free from bacterial growth.
   C. The lower small intestines and large intestines have a luxuriant growth of a number of species, including the Escherichia coli, some Clostridia species, Streptococcus fecalis and many anaerobic non-spore-forming bacilli (e.g. Bacteroides species). (Fecal material is composed largely of dead and living micro-organisms.)
   D. The remaining tissues of the body, including the blood, are normally free from micro-organisms.
   E. When normal flora are destroyed, pathogenic organisms may be able to grow and reproduce to a greater extent than usual.

Facts Pertaining to the Mode of Infections by Micro-organisms

1. Organisms may be transferred from the source to a new host directly by:

A. Contact with an infected part of the body or discharges which are infected.
B. Contaminated objects (fomites).

2. Organisms may be transferred from the source to a new host indirectly by:
   A. Air (particles of dust, droplets of moisture, droplet nuclei).
      (1) Coughing, sneezing, violent talking or laughing cause the expulsion of droplets of respiratory secretions into the air.
      (2) Effective air change by good ventilation decreases the number of droplet nuclei.
   B. Sewage.
   C. Milk. (Milk provides an excellent medium for microbial growth.)
   D. Food.
   E. Water.
   F. Vectors (including ticks, mites, lice, fleas, mosquitoes and flies).
3. Each communicable disease is transferred in one or more rather definite ways determined by:
   A. The way in which the pathogen leaves the source.
   B. The portal of entry of each type of pathogen.
   C. The ability of the pathogen to survive outside the host.

FACTS PERTAINING TO SPECIFIC PATHOGENIC BACTERIA

1. *Salmonella typhosa* causes typhoid fever.
   A. The organisms may be found in the urine, feces and blood. (Organisms may be found in the gall bladder, leaving the body through the feces, months and years after the acute disease is over.)
   B. The organisms may be transferred directly by fecal material, urine or blood and indirectly by contaminated food and water. (Flies may be responsible for indirect transmission.)
   C. The portal of entry is the mouth.
   D. The organisms can live in ice for as long as 3 months and in moist feces as long as 2 months.

2. Other species of Salmonella cause salmonellosis (including paratyphoid fever and food poisoning).
   A. The organisms may be found in feces and vomitus of infected human beings or animals.
   B. The organisms may be transferred directly by fecal material or vomitus and indirectly by contaminated food and water. (Flies may be responsible for indirect transmission.)
   C. The portal of entry is the mouth.
   D. The organisms can live outside of the host for weeks and possibly months.
3. Species of the genus Shigella cause bacillary dysentery.
   A. The organisms may be found in feces and vomitus.
   B. The organisms may be transferred directly by fecal material or vomitus and indirectly by contaminated food and water. (Flies are frequently responsible for indirect transmission.)
   C. The portal of entry is the mouth.
   D. The organisms can live outside of the host for weeks and possibly months.
4. The *Vibrio comma* causes cholera.
   A. The organisms may be found in feces and vomitus.
   B. The organisms may be transferred directly by fecal material or vomitus and indirectly by contaminated food and water.
   C. The portal of entry is the mouth.
5. Species of the genus Brucella cause brucellosis (undulant fever).
   A. The organisms may be found in cattle, goats and pigs.
   B. The organisms may be transferred directly by contact or indirectly by food products from the infected animals.
   C. The portals of entry are the mouth and the skin.
   D. The organisms can exist outside the host in milk and milk products or on the skins of animals. (Pasteurization of milk and milk products is an important control measure.)
6. *Pasteurella tularensis* causes tularemia.
   A. The organisms may be found in rabbits and other wild rodents and game birds. (In infected human beings the

organisms are found in infected lymph glands.)

B. The organisms may be transferred directly by contact with the skins of infected animals or indirectly by the bites of infected ticks, deer flies and other insects and by infected meat.

C. The portals of entry are the mouth and the skin.

D. The organisms can survive for some time in water and in dead bodies.

7. *Pasteurella pestis* causes plague.

A. The organisms may be found in rats and, in pneumonic plague, may be found in the respiratory tracts and in the urine and feces of infected persons.

B. The organisms may be transferred directly by respiratory discharges (in pneumonic plague) and by contact with infected animals and indirectly by rat fleas which are vectors.

C. The portals of entry may be the respiratory tract, the mouth and the skin.

8. *Hemophillus pertussis* causes pertussis (whooping cough).

A. The organisms are found in the upper respiratory tract and occasionally in the epithelium of the eye.

B. The organisms may be transferred directly by respiratory discharges and indirectly by air contaminated with droplets of respiratory discharges.

C. The portal of entry is the respiratory tract (nose and throat).

D. The organisms are not very resistant outside the host.

9. *Corynebacterium diphtheriae* causes diphtheria.

A. The organisms may be found in the upper respiratory tract and the skin.

B. The organisms may be transferred directly by respiratory discharges or from the skin and indirectly by air or milk contaminated by the micro-organisms.

C. The portal of entry is the respiratory tract (nose and throat) and, occasionally, the skin.

D. The organisms are strictly parasitic and are easily killed by heat and various chemicals.

10. *Neisseria meningitides* causes epidemic meningitis.
    A. The organisms are found in the nasopharynx, the blood, spinal fluid and skin petechiae.
    B. The organisms may be transferred directly by respiratory discharges (and blood or spinal fluid) and indirectly by air contaminated with droplets of respiratory discharges.
    C. The portal of entry is the respiratory tract (nose and throat).
    D. The organisms are fragile and can live only briefly outside of the host.
11. *Neisseria gonorrheae* causes gonorrhea.
    A. The organisms may be found in the genito-urinary tract, pelvic cavity, eye, heart or joints.
    B. The organisms may be transferred directly by contact with infected areas or by discharges from the genito-urinary tract, pelvic cavity or conjunctiva.
    C. The portals of entry are the mucous membrane of the genito-urinary tract and the conjunctiva.
    D. The organisms are fragile and die quickly when they are exposed to the air or are dried.
12. *Diplococcus pneumoniae* frequently causes pneumonia.
    A. The organisms may be found in the respiratory tract.
    B. The organisms may be transferred directly by respiratory discharges and indirectly by air contaminated with droplets of respiratory discharges.
    C. The portal of entry is the respiratory tract (nose and throat).
    D. The organisms are strictly parasitic and easily killed by heat and various chemicals.
13. Species of Streptococci cause scarlet fever, septic sore throat, upper respiratory infections, erysipelas and puerperal fever or may act as opportunists causing wound infections and infections of many body tissues (e.g. ear, lungs or kidneys).
    A. The organisms may be found:
       (1) In the respiratory tract during scarlet fever, septic sore throat, and various respiratory infections.
       (2) In the skin in erysipelas.

(3) In the uterus in puerperal fever.

(4) In the blood stream if the organisms invade blood vessels.

(5) In the drainage from infected wounds or infected body tissues.

B. The organisms may be transferred directly by discharges from infected parts of the body or indirectly by air, milk and milk products and food which have been contaminated with discharges.

C. The portals of entry may be the respiratory tract (nose and throat), the skin or the mucous membrane of the reproductive tract in women.

D. Streptococci are fairly resistant to drying and can live in milk and food for some time.

E. Streptococci are pyogenic organisms.

F. Some streptococci are usually present in the upper respiratory tract.

G. Animals (e.g. cows) may be infected with streptococci (e.g. in the udders).

14. *Staphylococcus aureus* (*Micrococcus pyogenes* var. aureus) can cause many types of infection (e.g. wound infections, skin infections or respiratory infections).

A. The organisms may be found on the skin and mucous membranes or wherever the infection exists.

B. The organisms may be transferred directly by contact or discharges from infected parts of the body.

C. The portals of entry may be the skin and mucous membranes, especially of the respiratory tract.

D. The staphylococci are hardy micro-organisms. (Many staphylococci become resistant to antibiotics.)

E. The organisms are pyogenic.

F. Virulent strains of staphylococci produce an exotoxin which can cause severe enteritis if ingested in sufficient quantity. The production of exotoxin may occur in poorly refrigerated foods (e.g. chopped meats or cream foods) which have been contaminated with the organisms.

15. The toxin formed by *Clostridium botulinum* causes botulism.

A. The organisms are saprophytes found in the soil.

B. The toxin is ingested with canned fruits and vegetables (the organisms grow best in a weakly acid to basic pH environment).

C. The organisms are anaerobic, gas-producing spore-formers.

16. The toxin produced by *Clostridium tetani* causes tetanus.
    A. The organisms are found normally in human and animal feces and in the soil as well as in the infected wounds when the individual has tetanus.
    B. The organisms may be transferred by contaminated soil.
    C. The portal of entrance is a wound in the skin (especially puncture wounds).
    D. The organisms are anaerobic spore-formers.
17. Several species of Clostridium (including *Clostridium perfringens*) cause gas gangrene.
    A. The organisms are normally found in human and animal feces and in the soil as well as in infected wounds when the individual has gas gangrene.
    B. The organisms may be transferred by contaminated soil.
    C. The portal of entry is a wound in the skin (especially deep or lacerated wounds).
    D. The organisms are anaerobic spore-formers.
18. *Mycobacterium tuberculosis* causes tuberculosis.
    A. The organisms are obligate parasites and may be found:
        (1) In man, in the respiratory tract (sometimes in the stomach if swallowed) or in body tissues which have been invaded by the organisms (e.g. meninges, lymph nodes, joints or skin).
        (2) In the cow, in the respiratory tract, the intestinal tract and in the udder.
    B. The portals of entry may be the respiratory tract or the gastro-intestinal tract.
    C. The organisms are capable of long survival inside or outside the host, particularly in sputum or pus. The organisms can remain encapsulated in the host (e.g. lungs or lymph glands) for many years.
19. *Treponema pallidum* causes syphilis.
    A. The organisms are obligate parasites and may be found:

(1) In the first stage of the disease, in the chancre.
(2) In the second stage of the disease, in lesions of the skin and mucous membranes.
(3) In the third stage of the disease, in various internal tissues.

B. The organisms may be transferred directly by contact (e.g. sexual intercourse, kissing) and may be transferred by an infected mother to an unborn child through the placenta.

C. The portals of entry may be the skin and mucous membranes.

D. The organisms are fragile and can live only very briefly outside the host.

20. Species of Borrelia and Fusobacterium cause Vincent's stomatitis, Vincent's gingivitis and Vincent's angina.
    A. These organisms are normally found in the mouths of human beings and may be considered to be secondary invaders when resistance is low.
    B. These organisms are not readily transferred from one person to another.

Facts Pertaining to Pathogenic Rickettsia

1. Rickettsia are obligate intracellular parasites and are natural parasites of arthropods such as fleas, lice, ticks, and mites.
2. Rickettsia are usually found in the alimentary canals of these arthropods. Rickettsia are generally introduced into the human host by injection into the skin (insect bites) or by the rubbing or scratching of skin contaminated with fecal material from the infected arthropod.
3. The animal reservoirs vary.
    A. Epidemic typhus is louse-borne and the animal reservoirs are human beings.
    B. Rocky Mountain Spotted Fever is tick-borne and there are various wild animal reservoirs.
    C. Q Fever is tick-borne and the animal reservoirs are primarily cattle and sheep. (In the transfer of these organisms, milk and air contaminated with dust from infected animals play important roles.)

Facts Pertaining to Pathogenic Viruses

1. Viruses are obligate intracellular parasites which cause specific communicable diseases, but may also cause infections in many tissues of the body following the specific disease process (e.g. encephalitis following mumps).
2. The virus of psittacosis is a natural parasite of many birds.
   A. The viruses can be found in bird droppings and dust containing bits of these droppings.
   B. The portal of entry is the respiratory tract (nose and throat).
3. The viruses of smallpox and chicken pox are found in the respiratory tract, in saliva and in the skin lesions.
   A. The viruses may be transferred directly by contact or by respiratory discharges and saliva.
   B. The portal of entry is usually the respiratory tract but may be the skin.
4. The virus of herpes simplex is in the tissues of infected persons (the virus generally remains there for life) and may be activated by a lowered resistance in the tissues.
   A. The virus may be transmitted by direct contact.
   B. The portal of entry is the skin or mucous membrane (generally of the face).
5. The virus of measles (Rubeola) is found in the respiratory tract.
   A. The organisms are transmitted directly by respiratory secretions.
   B. The portal of entry is in the respiratory tract (nose and throat).
6. The virus of German measles (Rubella) is found in the respiratory tract.
   A. The organisms are transmitted directly by respiratory secretions.
   B. The portal of entry is the respiratory tract (nose and throat).
7. The virus of infectious hepatitis is found in feces, blood, and, possibly, in the urine and naso-pharyngeal secretions.
   A. The viruses may be transmitted directly or indirectly by

food and water contaminated by feces and, possibly, urine and naso-pharyngeal secretions.

B. The portals of entry include the gastro-intestinal tract and possibly the respiratory tract.

8. The virus of serum hepatitis is found in the blood.
   A. The organisms are transmitted directly by blood.
   B. The portal of entry is usually the skin (through injection).
9. The virus of influenza is found in the respiratory tract.
   A. The organisms are transmitted directly by respiratory secretions and indirectly by air contaminated with droplets of respiratory secretions.
   B. The portal of entry is the respiratory tract (nose and throat).
10. The virus of the common cold is found in the respiratory tract.
    A. The organisms are usually transmitted directly by respiratory secretions or indirectly by air contaminated with droplets of respiratory secretions.
    B. The portal of entry is the respiratory tract (nose and throat).
11. The virus of the mumps is found in saliva.
    A. The organisms are usually transmitted directly.
    B. The portal of entry is the mouth.
12. Little is known about the virus which causes infectious mononucleosis, and the modes of transmission are unknown.
13. The virus of rabies is found in the saliva of infected animals (e.g. dogs, foxes, bats, skunks or cattle) and infected human beings.
    A. The organisms are transmitted directly by the saliva.
    B. The portal of entry is the broken skin (i.e. bites from infected animals).
14. The virus of poliomyelitis is found in the nasopharynx (early) and in the feces (from the onset of the disease up to a month or more).
    A. The organisms are usually transmitted directly by infective discharges, but contaminated food may provide an indirect means. (Flies may be an important means of transmission.)
    B. The portals of entry are the nose and throat.

15. The virus of encephalitis is found in birds and animals.
    A. The organisms are transmitted indirectly by arthropod vectors (e.g. mosquitoes).
    B. There is no evidence of person-to-person transmission.

Facts Pertaining to Pathogenic Fungi

1. Fungi can cause disease in persons of normal health but some of the common skin and mucous membrane fungous infections occur in people when tissues are injured by constant uncleanliness or abnormal moisture.
2. Saprophytic food-spoilage types and plant pathogens are only rarely associated with human disease.
3. The dermatophyte fungi causes dermatomycosis and may be found in the skin, hair or nails.
    A. The fungi are usually transmitted directly by contact.
    B. Pet animals are sometimes a source of some types of ringworm.
4. *Candida albicans* causes moniliasis.
    A. The organisms are found, normally, in mouths and in the feces.
    B. The organisms tend to develop in tissues injured by malnutrition or irritation, in tissues kept abnormally moist or in tissues whose normal flora have been reduced (e.g. by antibiotics).
5. *Histoplasma capsulatum* cause histoplasmosis.
    A. Suspected animal sources include rodents and pigeons.
    B. Spores can be found in water, air and in the soil around farm buildings.
    C. The organisms are not spread from man to man.
6. *Coccidiodes immitis* causes coccidiodomycosis.
    A. Rats, cattle, sheep and dogs may harbor the fungus.
    B. The fungus is present in soil and is spread by dust-borne spores.

Facts Pertaining to Pathogenic Protozoa

1. *Endameba histolytica* causes amebiasis.
    A. The source of the organisms is the feces of infected persons.

B. The cysts may be transmitted directly by feces and indirectly by food, water, and flies.
C. The trophozoites encyst in the intestines and the cysts are passed in formed stool.
D. The cysts become infective upon ingestion.
E. Cysts can survive several weeks outside a host, but are fairly susceptible to cold and drying.

2. Species of the genus Plasmodia cause malaria.
   A. The sources of the organisms are the blood of man and the saliva of the infected female Anopheles mosquito.
   B. The organisms are transmitted by bites of the infected female Anopheles mosquito.
   C. Malaria may be transmitted by blood transfusions from infected persons.
3. *Trichomonas vaginalis* causes trichomonas vaginitis.
   A. The sources are the vagina or urethra of women or the urethra of man.
   B. The organisms may be transmitted directly by contact or by fomites.
   C. It is not certain whether this protozoan is a true pathogen or an opportunist.

Facts Pertaining to Specific Helminth Infestations

1. The male and female pinworms live in the cecum.
   A. The gravid female migrates to the perineum where she lays her eggs.
   B. If the eggs are ingested, they hatch in the intestines and develop into adult worms.
   C. The eggs may be found on contaminated parts of the body, fomites, in dust particles and in the air.
2. The intestinal hookworms live in the small intestine.
   A. Eggs which are laid are passed in the feces.
   B. Larvae hatch from the eggs and grow in the soil.
   C. After approximately 7 days, the larvae are able to penetrate the skin of a new host.
   D. The larvae then pass through the blood to the respiratory tract, are swallowed and the adult forms develop in the small intestine.

3. The large intestinal roundworms cause ascariasis.
   A. The adult worms live in the intestinal tract.
   B. The female worm lays eggs which are passed in the feces.
   C. After about 3 weeks the eggs, if ingested (e.g. from contaminated food, drink or fingers), reach the intestines where the larvae are liberated.
   D. The larvae penetrate the intestinal mucosa and go, via the lymphatics, to the blood vessels and, by the circulation of the blood, reach the lungs.
   E. After reaching the lungs, the larvae migrate up the respiratory tract, are swallowed and develop into adult worms in the small intestines.
4. The trichina worm causes trichiniasis.
   A. The adult worms live in the intestinal tract.
   B. The females produce larvae which are capable of encysting in muscle tissue.
   C. Man contracts infestation by ingesting the flesh of carnivorous animals (e.g. hogs) which contain encysted larvae.
   D. The ingested larvae develop in the intestines and larvae produced by the female encyst in muscle tissue.
5. The source of tapeworms which infect man is man himself.
   A. The adult tapeworm lives in the small intestine and produces eggs which are passed through the feces.
   B. If animals ingest these eggs (e.g. steer, hogs or fish) the eggs develop in the small intestines, the developed embryo passes via the blood to muscles where it encysts.
   C. Viable encysted forms when ingested by man develop to adult forms in the small intestine.
   D. One type of tapeworm which infests man needs no intermediate host; the eggs are immediately infective for the same or another person.

Facts Pertaining to Immunity

1. Natural immunity seems to be due to the general defense mechanisms of the body.
2. Immunity to each specific disease of microbial origin is due to the presence of specific antibodies.

3. Active immunity may be acquired as a result of the development of specific antibodies from:
   A. The body's response to an actual attack of the disease.
   B. The body's response to the introduction of antigenic biologicals, including:
      (1) Living cultures.
      (2) Killed cultures.
      (3) Derivatives of cultures.
4. There is usually prolonged immunity to the following diseases:
   A. Cholera, plague, diphtheria, scarlet fever, typhoid fever and paratyphoid fever.
   B. Rocky Mountain spotted fever and typhus.
   C. Chicken pox, small pox, measles, mumps and pertussis.
5. There is little if any immunity developed with the following diseases:
   A. Erysipelas, gonorrhea, syphilis and pneumonia.
   B. Common cold, herpes simplex and influenza.
6. Antigenic biologicals available for immunication against specific diseases include those for the following diseases:
   A. Smallpox. (Many state and local governments require vaccination.)
   B. Pertussis, tetanus, diphtheria and poliomyelitis. (Immunization is recommended early in life.)
   C. Typhoid, paratyphoid, cholera, epidemic typhus, tuberculosis, Rocky Mountain spotted fever, influenza, some types of streptococcal infection and rabies.
      (1) Immunizations may be recommended (or required) when the possibility of infection is increased by such factors as occupation, environmental conditions and actual exposure.
      (2) BCG vaccine is available as immunization against tuberculosis and is believed to have some usefulness.
7. There are some biological preparations which can be used in the skin to test for immunity or hypersensitivity developed by previous exposure to certain diseases. These tests include:
   A. The Schick test and Maloney test for diphtheria.
   B. The Dick test for scarlet fever.

C. The tuberculin test for tuberculosis (Mantoux test or Vollmer patch test).

D. The Histoplasmin test for histoplasmosis.

E. The Coccidiodin test for coccidiodomycosis.

8. Passive immunity may be acquired temporarily by the introduction of antibodies into the body.

A. Immune sera (e.g. gamma globulin for measles) may be injected.

B. A fetus in utero receives antibodies from the mother's blood.

CHAPTER IV: *Social Science Principles and Hypotheses and Related Nursing Care*

SEVERAL points need to be emphasized before the reader gives consideration to the material presented in the balance of this chapter. It cannot be stressed often enough that *the material is not a complete outline of social science principles important to nursing*. The material does represent those factors which were important in a number of actual patient-nurse situations. As such, they can be used as a starting point for further determination of important concepts and principles. Many of the statements lead quite logically to additional information which the nurse might need in order to give effective patient care. For example, in Section A, I-D, we find the statement, "Any attempt on the part of external forces to remove or destroy an individual's psychological defenses against anxiety will cause an increase in the anxiety experienced by the individual." This statement is of little value to the nurse unless she knows what these mechanisms are and the dynamics of how they operate in the patient's defense. Only four specific mechanisms are mentioned in the substatements in Section A because of the data limitations. A logical elaboration would include other important mechanisms.

It is of particular interest to note that Section C, regarding human needs, is the most extensively developed of the five sections. This is due to the exceedingly large number of situations reported which described patient distress or satisfaction in the area of comfort and security, as associated with need-satisfaction. Within this area, the most important single factor was the patient's need to cope successfully with a current situation; to know what was happening, what was expected of him and what action was required to resolve current problems. Second in importance was the patient's need for a situational definition—the need to know who and where he was and how he and others fitted into the current environmental picture. These two needs were demonstrated repeatedly in the incidents reported, and the extensive development of sub-principles and hypotheses represent the wide variety of situations in which these needs were depicted.

It should be pointed out that, even with the condensation of statements which took place in the process of organization, there is still considerable overlapping and repetition. This is unfortunate from the standpoint of reviewing the material, but is probably unavoidable.

It might be helpful to the reader to remember that the incidents were collected from only medical, surgical and obstetrical services. Some interesting speculations might be made, considering the omission of such services as pediatrics and psychiatry. For example, would there have been a much larger number of statements in Section A, regarding personality integration and growth and development, if pediatrics had been included, or in Section B, regarding behavior manifestations, if psychiatry had been included? Also, what significance can we attach to the fact that there were no remarkable differences in the kinds of incidents and resulting statements as drawn from medical, surgical and obstetrical areas?

The material is organized in five major sections, the first four of which being concerned with single conceptual statements. At the end of each section are found examples of related nursing care. The nursing care statements are intended to demonstrate examples of how social science knowledge can be used by the nurse to make judgments and decisions in giving patient care. Again, this area is incomplete, since it intends only to provide examples of nursing applications of science principles.

A further word of explanation needs to be said regarding Section E. In the process of analysis there were occasional incidents which demonstrated patient harm or benefit as a result of nursing action, but which did not contain sufficient information to arrive at basic science statements. For these situations, the action-guiding statements were made in terms of nursing principles. Of course, these principles could be traced ultimately to some basic science knowledge, but not on the basis of evidence contained in the described incident. It was felt that, even without the basic science to accompany the statement, these nursing principles were sufficiently important to be retained and used as guides to nursing action.

No attempt was made to designate the specific social science areas (i.e., psychology, sociology, anthropology) to which the concepts, principles and hypotheses were most closely related. A cursory glance at the material would seem to indicate that the majority of the statements are most likely to be related to psychology. A closer look reveals the interrelatedness of all three of the major social science areas in the development of the four conceptual statements. Perhaps this interdependence and overlapping has some implications for methods of teaching nursing students the application of principles.

The balance of this chapter contains the complete material resulting from the analysis of the incidents. It is presented in outline form for the sake of clarity and brevity.

SECTION A

Social Science Principles and Hypotheses and Related Nursing Care for the Concept:

"Individual psychological equilibrium requires the maintenance of an adequately functioning integrated organism."

I

SOCIAL SCIENCE PRINCIPLES AND HYPOTHESES

1. Psychological equilibrium requires the ability to perceive clearly and interpret internal and external data.
   A. Adequacy of perception of a situation may require utilization of one or several of the senses, depending upon the situation.
   B. The perception of a situation is to some extent unique for each individual in the situation.
   C. An individual will react to a situation or event as he perceives it, regardless of the reality of the situation (or how the majority of other people see the situation).
   D. Perception is influenced by a variety of internal and external factors.
      (1) What an individual perceives in a given situation is influenced by his past experiences, his present interests, and his physiological and psychological condition.
      (2) An individual who misinterprets situations or events will react to these situations as he interprets them.
      (3) The preconceptions an individual has about a situation or another person will influence his reaction and behavior in relation to that situation or person.
      (4) Some individuals are hypersensitive to environmental events.

(5) The individual who is hypersensitive to sensory stimuli (environmental events) will tend to react to stimulation regardless of need for rest.

(6) Preoccupation with personal matters, concentration of attention on environmental stimuli, and other distracting influences will interfere with adequate perception of a situation.

2. Psychological equilibrium requires that the individual have an adequate means for communicating with others and/or for self-expression.

A. Communication between individuals takes place in a variety of ways.

(1) Non-verbal behavior is an essential part of the communication process.

(2) The use of mutually understood symbols is a prerequisite for effective communication.

(3) Every culture provides symbolic means for communication between individuals and groups of individuals.

B. Communication is influenced by a variety of internal and external factors.

(1) Communication between individuals is influenced by the relationship which exists between the individuals involved in communication.

(2) Symbols of communication are interpreted by the individual in the light of the situation in which he finds himself and according to his unique background of experience.

(3) Preoccupation with personal matters, concentration of attention on environmental events, and other distracting influences will interfere with effective communication.

(a) The introduction or occurrence of thoughts regarding an emotionally charged subject may interfere with an individual's ability to communicate effectively.

(b) Extremes of emotion are likely to interfere with the ability to communicate.

C. Expression of feeling or emotion may be achieved in a variety of ways.

(1) Feelings which cannot be directly expressed toward the object or individual engendering the feelings may be displaced onto other objects or individuals.

(2) Illness and/or physical symptoms (physiological phenomena) may be used as a method of expressing unconscious feeling.

(3) Crying may be an effective form of behavior for relieving tension or expressing emotion which cannot be otherwise expressed.

(4) Verbalization of problems which are causing tension in the presence of a non-judgmental but receptive listener will often be helpful in temporarily reducing the tensions caused by the problem.

3. Psychological equilibrium is influenced by intellectual functioning.

A. In general, psychological equilibrium is enhanced if the individual is able to think clearly and rationally.

(1) For an individual who is confused, frequent re-orientation by those coming into his environment may be helpful in decreasing the confusion and the attendant fears caused by the confused state.

(2) The attention span of the confused person is usually short and easily interrupted.

(3) Extremes of emotion may interfere with rational behavior, learning processes and clear thinking.

(4) The physical environment has a substantial influence on an individual's emotional reaction and intellectual functioning.

(5) An individual's physiological state has an influence on psychological functioning.

(6) An individual's psychological state has an influence on physiological functioning.

(7) An individual who has delusions will act on the basis of the delusions regardless of the apparent reality of a situation or any attempts to convince him of the falsity of his ideas.

B. A person's psychological reactions (ideas, beliefs, convictions) can cause the subjective experiencing of physiological symptoms where no physiological pathology can be demonstrated.

4. Psychological equilibrium requires the development of and ability to utilize psychological mechanisms for warding off anxiety and for adequate adaptation to life situations.
   A. Any attempt on the part of external forces to remove or destroy an individual's psychological defenses against anxiety will cause an increase in the anxiety experienced by the individual.
   B. Unconscious anxiety may be dissipated through projection of unconscious feelings onto the external environment.
   C. Feelings which cannot be directly expressed toward the object or individual engendering the feeling may be displaced toward other objects or individuals.
   D. Several psychological mechanisms (such as identification and incorporation) may be utilized by the individual in successfully relating to others without anxiety.
   E. The mechanism of identification is utilized in learning role and function in life situations.
5. Psychological equilibrium requires that the individual have and be able to utilize the ability and opportunity for learning.
   A. A behavior which provides an adequate response (reduces a need) in one situation is likely to be repeated in similar situations.
   B. Effective learning depends upon adequate communication between teacher and learner.
   C. Motivation is prerequisite to optimum learning. (A person who is not motivated will demonstrate only minimal new learning.)
      (1) Comfort in the learning situation is increased if motivation for learning is positive (rewarding) rather than negative.
      (2) Change in behavior may be motivated by the anticipation of desirable conditions which will result from the behavior.

D. Learning is influenced by a variety of internal and external factors.

(1) Individual differences have a substantial influence on learning (what is learned, rate of learning, etc.).

(2) Learning is more likely to be effective if the learner has the opportunity to try out the new behavior to be learned.

(3) Repeated performance is necessary to the acquisition of a complicated motor skill.

(4) Learning is facilitated when an individual sees the relationship between what he is learning and his personal needs and problems.

(5) Disturbing emotional factors may interfere with effective learning.

(a) Disturbing emotional factors may interfere with perception of situations and with the execution of behavior.

(b) In extremely tense or traumatic situations an individual may need frequent repetition of what is to be learned or repeated successful experiences before learning can take place.

(6) What a person learns in any given situation depends upon what he perceives.

(7) The acquisition of new behavior is partially dependent upon the individual's physiological and psychological readiness to learn.

(8) If an individual is able to recognize or experience for himself what he is able to do, learning is likely to be more effective.

6. Psychological equilibrium requires adequate integration of all aspects of the individual's personality.

A. A person whose methods of adaptation are flexible will adjust to life situations with greater ease and satisfaction than one whose methods are rigid.

B. Adequate personality integration requires that an individual participate with and be accepted by other individuals and groups of individuals.

(1) Adequate personality integration requires that an

individual be able to identify with other individuals.

(2) Adequate personality integration requires that the individual have the opportunity to learn and subsequently achieve satisfaction in practicing socio-cultural roles.

(a) The child develops familiarity with role and status expectations through social interaction.

(b) One of the methods by which individuals learn the socio-cultural limits for behavior is through identification with other individuals in the environment.

(c) One of the methods by which the individual learns the socio-cultural limits for behavior is through "reality testing."

C. Individual personality is partially determined by the culture within which growth and maturation takes place.

D. Adequate personality integration requires some degree of satisfaction of the basic primary and acquired needs. (See Section C for statements concerning specific needs and need satisfaction.)

II

NURSING CARE RELATED TO THE PRINCIPLES AND HYPOTHESES

1. "Psychological equilibrium requires the ability to perceive clearly and interpret internal and external data." The nurse can assist the patient to maintain clarity of perception and correctness in interpretation by:

A. Increasing her knowledge and understanding of the individual patient and his life in order to anticipate how he will perceive a specific situation.

B. Attempting to determine and provide factual information the patient may need for clarity of perception of a situation.

C. Prevention of factors which might cause misconceptions or interferences in clarity of perception. To achieve this the nurse can:

(1) Increase her awareness of how her own behavior might be interpreted by the patient, with subsequent control of her behavior to prevent misconceptions.
(2) Insure simplicity and a minimum of perceptual experiences for the confused person or others who might have perceptual handicaps.
(3) Decrease environmental stimuli for the person who is hypersensitive to such stimuli.
(4) Remove or control distracting influences which might interfere with clarity of perception.
(5) Provide repeated perceptual experiences for the individual who has some physiological or psychological handicap or interference with clarity of perception.

D. Providing opportunities for sensory perception of situations which are of concern to the patient.
E. Attempting to determine clarity of perception by questioning, asking for a repeat of information, etc.
F. Providing information or perceptual experiences which the patient will be able to interpret according to his own background of experiences.
G. Attempting to determine and correct misconceptions.
H. Carefully considering factors in the patient's life situation, including psychological and physiological factors, in order to anticipate how he will perceive a specific situation.
I. Providing clarifying explanation or interpretation of data in situations where clarity of perception is limited by lack of understanding.

2. "Psychological equilibrium requires that the individual have an adequate means for communicating with others and/or for self-expression." The nurse can help the patient in maintaining effective communication and in achieving satisfactory expression by:

A. Providing an opportunity for the patient to talk with appropriate persons regarding subjects of concern and interest to him.
B. Increasing her mastery of language symbols, within reason,

so that she can understand what the patient is trying to communicate.

C. Talking to the patient in language which he can understand.

D. Increasing her ability to interpret non-verbal communications so that the patient may be understood.

E. Utilizing non-verbal behavior to communicate with the patient.

F. Controlling environmental factors which may interfere with the patient's communication.

G. Providing for or insuring a relationship with someone which is conducive to effective communication. This may be accomplished by:

(1) Assignment of personnel over a period of time to allow the patient to know someone well enough to feel free to talk with them about personal subjects of concern.

(2) Demonstration of an attitude of acceptance or non-judgment on the part of the listener when the patient is expressing ideas, attitudes, feelings, etc.

(3) Awareness of her own attitude and behavior which might prevent the patient from communicating freely.

(4) Control of her own behavior to prevent using the patient as a listener.

(5) The demonstration of attitudes and behaviors which indicate interest in what the patient may have to say and concern for his welfare.

(6) Indicating by words and behavior that she understands what the patient is trying to communicate.

H. Assisting the patient to clarify ideas, attitudes, etc. by asking for clarification without implying the desirability or undesirability of a specific idea, attitude, etc.

I. Avoiding attempts to communicate important information when the patient is emotionally disturbed or distracted.

J. Repetition of important information when there is some existing interference with communication, such as emotional disturbance, distraction, temporary physical or mental disability.

K. Providing a means of non-verbal communication when there is some handicap in the area of verbal communication.

L. Keeping her communications clear and simple, especially when there is some interference with clarity of perception.

M. Encouraging expression of negative (socially censured) feelings in a non-harmful situation when such expression will be therapeutic. This implies:
   (1) Non-judgment by the listener.
   (2) Insurance of no retaliation as a result of expression of feeling.
   (3) Protection of the patient from attitudes of others who might be judgmental or retaliatory.

N. Provision of a means for expressing negative (socially censured) feelings in a non-verbal way when verbal expression is either not desirable, not possible, or insufficient to decrease accumulated tension caused by the feelings. This implies:
   (1) Allowing or encouraging the patient to cry without resulting feelings of inadequacy or non-acceptance.
   (2) Providing physical activity which will dissipate tension.
   (3) Remaining calm, non-judgmental and non-restrictive when the patient displays aggressive or hostile behavior when such behavior is non-harmful to others.

O. Assisting the patient to develop more effective means of communication and expression when current means may be harmful or ineffective.

P. Assisting with clarification of communication or increasing the opportunity for communication between the patient and others in the environment.

3. "Psychological equilibrium is influenced by intellectual functioning." The nurse can assist the patient effectively to utilize mental faculties by:

A. Controlling the environment to prevent confusion or additional confusion whenever possible.

B. Assisting the patient to think constructively. This implies:
   (1) Asking thought-provoking questions.

(2) Maintaining a supportive attitude while the patient verbally works through problems.
(3) Providing needed information.

C. Controlling the environment, including her own behavior, to prevent or remove emotionally disturbing factors which might interfere with rational thinking and behavior. This implies:
(1) Prevention or removal of anxiety or fear-producing factors.
(2) Prevention or removal of distracting influences.
(3) Making the patient physically comfortable through physical care and control of the environment.

D. Providing external control of the patient's behavior while he is unable to maintain rational control himself.

E. Providing assistance as necessary for psycho-social adjustment when the patient is unable to use intellectual faculties. This implies:
(1) Giving simple directions the patient can follow even when he may not be able to understand the reasons for the action.
(2) Providing written or verbal information or directions as needed when the patient is unable to remember over a period of time.
(3) Protecting the patient from subsequent embarrassment due to inability to control his behavior.
(4) Protecting the patient by guiding or controlling his behavior when his judgment is impaired.
(5) Providing for the satisfaction of the patient's needs when impairment of mental faculties prevent him from taking independent action to satisfy his own needs.

4. "Psychological equilibrium requires the development of and ability to utilize psychological mechanisms for warding off anxiety and for adequate adaptation to life situations." The nurse can assist the patient toward adjustment in this area by:

A. Increasing her awareness and acceptance of psychological mechanisms the patient might be using.

B. Controlling her own behavior to prevent destruction of the psychological mechanisms the patient may be utilizing whenever the patient's adequate adjustment is dependent upon these mechanisms.

C. Accepting or encouraging the use of constructive and/or socially approved mechanisms whenever the situation indicates.

5. "Psychological equilibrium requires that the individual have and be able to utilize the ability and opportunity for learning." The nurse can assist the patient in this area by:

A. Determining or recognizing the patient's specific learning needs.

B. Utilizing principles of learning to assist the patient in his learning tasks. (See statements under Section I; Social Science Principles and Hypotheses, part 5.)

6. "Psychological equilibrium requires adequate integration of all aspects of the individual's personality." The nurse can assist the patient in this area by:

A. Helping him to gain a realistic perception of himself, especially in situations where he is undergoing changes in self-concept as a result of illness or hospitalization.

B. Demonstrating, through attitudes and behavior, that she accepts him as a worthwhile individual without judgment, or attempts to "reform," so long as his behavior is nonharmful.

C. Giving the patient psychological support as he adapts to his role in the hospital social structure.

D. Assisting the patient in the satisfaction of his basic needs insofar as they are disturbed by the primary cause of hospitalization and/or resulting from hospitalization.

SECTION B

Social Science Principles and Hypotheses and Related Nursing Care for the Concept:

"All behavior is a function of the relationships between specifiable antecedent events."

I

SOCIAL SCIENCE PRINCIPLES AND HYPOTHESES

1. Some kinds of behavior may be identified as common human reactions inherent to the nature of the organism.
   A. All human needs are interrelated; a disturbance in one area of function will cause reciprocal reactions in other areas of function.
      (1) The human organism responds physiologically to emotionally disturbing situations or experiences.
      (2) The human organism responds psychologically to physiologically disturbing situations or experiences.
      (3) Persistent lack of satisfaction of psychological needs appears to be correlated with physiological reactions.
      (4) Persistent lack of satisfaction of physiological needs appears to be correlated with psychological reactions.
      (5) Psychological comfort and well-being are partially dependent upon physiological comfort and well-being.
      (6) Physiological comfort and well-being are partially dependent upon psychological comfort and well-being.
   B. Psychotic behavior may be beyond the conscious control of the individual exhibiting that behavior.

C. Sleep and relaxation are more likely to occur under conditions of reduced anxiety.

D. Physical symptoms may arise from psychogenic origins, independent of objectively demonstrable physiological pathology.

E. A person's beliefs, ideas, convictions, etc., can cause the person to experience subjective physiological symptoms where no physiological pathology can be demonstrated.

F. An individual's attitudes and beliefs influence his behavioral response.

G. An individual's mental or emotional state consciously and unconsciously influences his behavior.

H. Distracting one's attention from anxiety-producing material or an anxiety-producing situation may reduce the anxiety felt in relation to the material or the situation.

2. Patterns of behavior are learned in the process of growth and development.

A. An individual may come to depend upon hostility, dependence, withdrawal, etc., as a method for handling problematic situations.

B. An individual is often likely to respond in a manner similar to the one by which he is approached.

C. A behavior which provides an adequate response (reduces a need) in one situation is likely to be repeated in similar situations.

D. An individual's reaction to a new situation is partially determined by his past experiences in similar situations.

E. Any given activity may be considered normal or healthy in one situation and abnormal or unhealthy in another situation, dependent upon cultural definition.

3. Some forms of behavior are specific indications of psychological disequilibrium from specific causes.

A. An individual who is threatened by interpersonal situations may tend to withdraw from social interaction in order to prevent or avoid greater psychological discomfort.

B. An individual who is in a state of gross disequilibrium will be more likely to experience an exaggerated emotional response to minor environmental disturbances than will the individual whose equilibrium is relatively stable.

C. Regressive behavior is a common reaction to physical illness.

D. An attitude of suspicion, doubt or mistrust may be an indication of underlying anxiety or insecurity.

E. An individual will experience feelings of inferiority or inadequacy if he is unable to live up to personal or social expectations.

F. An abrupt change of subject may indicate an area which is emotionally charged or painful.

G. Undesirable forms of behavior may indicate an individual's need for and attempts to obtain a positive response from others.

4. Some forms of behavior are non-specific indications of a disturbance of psychological equilibrium, the causes of which must be determined by further investigation.

A. Any disturbance of psychological equilibrium will cause a primary reaction of anxiety, fear, apprehension or tension.

(1) Many forms of behavior may be utilized by the individual in his attempts to remove, escape from or obliterate the discomfort of overt anxiety, fear, apprehension or tension.

(2) Anxiety is commonly accompanied by physical reactions such as tremor, loss of appetite, perspiration, sleeplessness, etc.

B. Attempts to manipulate or control the external environment (in excess of the control necessary for safety) may be an indication of an individual's attempt to dissipate or alleviate anxiety.

C. Illogical or irrational behavior may result from extremes of fear or anxiety.

D. Excessive demands for attention may indicate psychological disequilibrium.

E. Regressive behavior may be an indication of underlying anxiety or emotional trauma.

F. Excessive complaints or dissatisfaction in a situation may be an indication of underlying anxiety.

G. Hostility may be a reaction to:
   (1) threats to the integrity of the organism.
   (2) frustration.
   (3) emotional stress.

H. Withdrawal from the environmental situation may be a reaction to:
   (1) frustration.
   (2) traumatic experiences in interpersonal relations.
   (3) threats to the integrity of the organism.

I. Illness and/or physical symptoms (physiological phenomena) may be used as a method of
   (1) gaining attention.
   (2) responding to a crisis situation.
   (3) expressing unconscious feeling or conflict.

J. Activities which are primarily used to meet physical needs (e.g., eating) may be used as a symbolic means for attaining emotional satisfaction, or in an attempt to resolve unconscious problems.

K. Atypical or, to the observer, unexpected behavior may indicate disequilibrium in some area of the organism's function.

II

NURSING CARE RELATED TO THE PRINCIPLES AND HYPOTHESES *

1. The ultimate goal of health care requires that the nurse be able to observe and report data regarding disturbances of psychological, psycho-biological and psycho-social equilibrium.

   A. In order to make meaningful observations the nurse must

* Knowledge and understanding of information contained in Section I, *Social Science Principles and Hypotheses,* help to achieve the goals as stated under *Related Nursing Care,* parts 1 and 2. Part 3 of *Related Nursing Care* provides examples for further utilization of the information contained in the principles section.

be able to identify behaviors which indicate disturbances of equilibrium.

B. In order to make meaningful observations the nurse must be able to correctly perceive and interpret the patient's verbal and non-verbal communications.

C. In order to make meaningful observations the nurse must purposefully observe the specific patient according to known possible causes of disturbance in the patient's life situation, in addition to general observations.

D. In order to make meaningful observations the nurse must be able to utilize principles of interviewing to elicit additional information. In so doing, the nurse must use judgment to avoid upsetting, disturbing or causing psychological trauma to the patient.

E. In order to report meaningful data, the nurse must be able to communicate effectively with other members of the health team.

2. The ultimate goals of health care require that the health team be able to analyze and interpret the observed data. (In this and the following statements, the health team includes the nurse.)

A. In order to meaningfully analyze and interpret the observed data, health team members must compare and contrast the patient's usual or expected behavior with his current behavior.

B. In order to meaningfully analyze and interpret the observed data health team members must be able to interpret the significance of a given form of behavior as it is displayed by the patient.

C. In order to meaningfully analyze and interpret the observed data, health team members must be able to determine the relationship of the patient's behavior to factors in his current life situation.

D. In order to meaningfully analyze and interpret the observed data, health team members must be able to compare and contrast the patient's behavior with known facts about the normal and abnormal psychology of behavior and function of the human organism.

E. In order to meaningfully analyze and interpret the observed data, health team members must draw conclusions regarding the source or sources of disturbance or dissatisfaction.

F. In order to meaningfully analyze and interpret the observed data, health team members must attempt to identify the socio-cultural factors which might influence the specific patient's behavioral reaction.

3. The ultimate goals of health care require that health team members be able to utilize knowledge and understanding of human behavior in responding to the patient in a therapeutic manner.

A. "All human needs are interrelated; a disturbance in one area of function will cause reciprocal reactions in other areas of function." The nurse can utilize this knowledge by:

(1) Making an effort to prevent or alleviate emotional disturbances which might interfere with the patient's progress toward health.

(2) Providing emotional support for the patient who is living through a traumatic experience.

(3) Assisting the patient, as feasible, in the satisfaction of physiological and psychological needs.

(4) Attempting to assist the patient toward physiological and psychological comfort when such efforts are consistent with the ultimate goals of health care for the individual.

B. "Psychotic behavior may be beyond the conscious control of the individual exhibiting that behavior." The nurse can utilize this knowledge by:

(1) Providing for external control of the patient's behavior if such behavior would be harmful to the patient or others.

(2) Protecting the patient from physiological or psychological damage from the environment, including other people in the environment.

(3) Maintaining an attitude of kindliness and acceptance

of the individual patient, even when his behavior must be controlled.

C. "Sleep and relaxation are more likely to occur under conditions of reduced anxiety." The nurse can utilize this knowledge by:
   (1) Attempting to avoid or alleviate anxiety producing situations when they interfere with needed sleep and rest.
   (2) Utilizing nursing measures and orders for medications to produce sleep and rest when anxiety is present and cannot be directly reduced.

D. "An individual's attitudes and beliefs influence his behavioral response." The nurse can utilize this knowledge by:
   (1) Attempting to plan nursing care, when feasible and desirable, in accord with the patient's attitudes and beliefs.
   (2) Assisting the patient to understand the goals of health care, and possibly assisting the patient to change attitudes and beliefs about health care, when such attitudes and beliefs are interfering with his progress toward health.

E. "An individual's mental or emotional state consciously and unconsciously influences his behavior." The nurse can utilize this knowledge by:
   (1) Attempting to alleviate mental and emotional states which might interfere with health goals.
   (2) Increasing her efforts to provide psychological support for the patient when his current mental or emotional state is causing distress.
   (3) Attempting to increase her effectiveness as a health team member by increasing her understanding of how her own behavior is influenced by her attitudes, beliefs, mental and emotional state.

SECTION C

Social Scence Principles and Hypotheses and Related Nursing Care for the Concept:

"There are some psychological and psycho-social needs which may be considered common to all people and for which there must be some degree of satisfaction if the individual is to maintain psychological or psycho-social equilibrium."

I

SOCIAL SCIENCE PRINCIPLES AND HYPOTHESES

1. In order to achieve and maintain psychological equilibrium, man must have satisfying relationships with other human beings, both individually and in groups.
   A. The feeling of being cared for or about by another person or persons is necessary for psychological homeostasis.
      (1) The attitudes and actions of others which indicate that the individual is worthy of attention, assistance or concern contributes to a feeling of being cared for or about.
      (2) The physical presence of those who are affectionally close reassures the individual that he is cared for.
   B. The awareness that one is not alone is basic to psychological homeostasis.
      (1) The sharing of experiences with others decreases the individual's feelings of aloneness.
      (2) The knowledge that one's behavior, experiences, feelings, etc., are not unique (are shared by others) decreases feelings of aloneness.
      (3) Effective interraction and communication with other individuals decreases the feeling of aloneness.

(4) The feeling that one is understood by others decreases the sense of aloneness.

C. The approval of others in one's socio-cultural environment is necessary for psychological homeostasis for the average person.

(1) Approval from others may be elicited by contributing valued actions, materials, beliefs or otherwise conforming to group standards.

(2) A feeling of being approved by others is achieved by being regarded or reacted to with positive as opposed to negative attitudes, with the value of the attitude being determined by the culture in which one lives.

(3) A feeling of being approved by others is increased if one's presence or participation in social groups is sought after.

D. Acceptance of one's self and one's individual differences by others is necessary for psychological homeostasis for the average person.

(1) The feeling that one is understood by others contributes to the feeling of being accepted.

(2) Inclusion as a participating member of social groups contributes to an individual's feeling of being accepted.

(3) Recognition and acceptance of one's individual differences by others contributes to the feeling of being accepted.

E. In order to experience satisfying relationships with others, the average individual must be able to feel that he will not be harmed as a result of the relationship.

(1) If an individual experiences a feeling of acceptance and esteem in relation to other individuals or groups of individuals, he will be better able to tolerate criticism or correction from this group or individual with a minimum of discomfort.

(2) In general, opportunities for satisfying relationships with others are increased if the individual is able to see others as trustworthy and capable.

(a) Trust and confidence in others are acquired through experiences in which the individual is not harmed or by which he has benefited.

(b) Trust and confidence in others are enhanced by the demonstration of concern and interest of others in the individual's welfare.

(3) An individual who is suspicious, fearful or distrustful of others may be threatened by interpersonal relations and may be unable to experience security and satisfaction in group relations until fear is decreased.

(4) Individuals who are threatened by interpersonal relations can achieve satisfaction and comfort in group relations by learning, through experience, that they will not be harmed in such situations.

F. The achievement of satisfying relationships with others is influenced by the psycho-biological structure and function of the organism.

(1) An individual's relationships with others are influenced by his perceptual ability and learned patterns of perception.

(a) An individual's relationships with others are influenced by his perception of his own role and the role of others in such relationships.

(b) The achievement of satisfactory relationships with others depends upon the ability to examine and evaluate one's own behavior in relation to others.

(c) The achievement of satisfactory relationships with others depends upon the ability to perceive oneself correctly and upon one's own capabilities and limitations.

(2) An individual's relationships with others are influenced by his self-concept and individual ego function.

(a) Positive self-esteem contributes to the achievement of satisfactory relationships with others.

(b) The ability to accept one's self and one's own capabilities and limitations contributes to the achievement of satisfactory relationships with others.

(c) Any mutilation or basic change in body structure will influence the individual's concept of himself and his relationships with others.

(3) Satisfying relationships with others depend upon the ability to communicate effectively.

G. The achievement of satisfying relationships with others is influenced by socio-cultural factors.

(1) If satisfactory interpersonal relationships are to be achieved and maintained, there must be a mutual recognition of culturally established roles, with behavior appropriate to these roles. (See Section D)

(2) In every society/culture there are established rules and codes of conduct to which the individual must adhere in order to be approved and accepted by others. (See Section D)

(3) In order to live comfortably within a given socio-cultural structure an individual must have the ability and opportunity to learn the accepted roles, rules and codes of conduct.

(a) One of the methods by which individuals learn the socio-cultural limits for behavior is through identification with other individuals in the environment.

(b) One of the methods by which individuals learn the socio-cultural limits for behavior is through "reality testing" (testing and exploration of the environment to determine results of specific behaviors).

(c) Personal definition and acceptance of a social role is learned through contact with the social environment in which the individual has the opportunity to see and practice the designated role.

(d) One of the methods by which individuals learn the socio-cultural limits for behavior is by having authority figures impose and enforce these limits.

(e) One of the ways in which society enforces the learning and practice of acceptable behavior is through a system of reward and punishment.

(4) A single individual may function in a variety of roles, depending upon the socio-cultural situation he happens to be in.

2. The achievement and maintenance of psychological equilibrium is enhanced if the individual has a sense of self-esteem.

A. Satisfying relationships with others are necessary to the development and maintenance of self-esteem.

B. The development and maintenance of self-esteem are dependent upon one's ability to function in accordance with the internalized standards, beliefs and values which have been acquired from the socio-cultural environment.

(1) In our culture, self-direction and independent action are highly valued forms of behavior.

(2) In some cultures, maintenance of individuality is necessary for a sense of self-esteem.

(3) A sense of self-esteem may be increased or decreased, depending upon one's identification with a particular socio-cultural group and the status of that group within the total social structure.

3. In order to achieve and maintain psychological equilibrium, the individual must have an adequate means of self-definition and situational definition. (He must know, to his own satisfaction, who he is, what his goals are.)

A. A sense of personal identity may be enhanced by the recognition (by oneself and others) of the person's individuality in relation to others.

B. Adequate personal and situational definition requires a knowledge and understanding of what the individual perceives to be the facts about himself and the situation.

(1) Knowledge of the facts about a situation requires sensory perception (seeing, hearing, touching, etc.) of factors in the situation.

(2) In addition to factual knowledge about a situation, an individual may be helped to achieve an adequate

personal and situational definition through beliefs and convictions which he holds to be true. (For some individuals, a belief in a supreme being or deity provides a means of personal and situational definition.)

C. Adequate self-definition is partially achieved through an individual's identification and sharing of experiences with other individuals and/or socio-cultural groups.

D. Adequate personal and situational definition requires clarity of perception of the individual's role and status in relation to others.

E. Adequate situational definition requires that the individual be aware of the behavioral limits of the situation.

F. Development and maintenance of an adequate personal and situational definition requires the establishment of familiar and consistent socio-cultural patterns.

(1) For some individuals, the possession of material objects provides a symbolic means of identification.

(2) Any mutilation or basic change in body structure will influence the individual's concept of himself and/or his relationship to others.

4. In order to establish and maintain psychological equilibrium, the average individual will attempt to achieve a feeling of safety and comfort in life situations.

A. A feeling of safety and comfort is engendered if the individual feels he is able to cope with life situations successfully. (i.e., control the situation and himself in such a way as to prevent harm.)

(1) The ability to handle life situations in a socially approved manner requires a knowledge of and ability to act within the socio-cultural limits of the situation.

(2) The ability to handle life situations with success is most probable when there is perception of the factors inherent in the situation, including the goal to be reached.

(a) One of the factors contributing to clarity of perception of a situation is possession of factual knowledge about the situation.

(b) Clarity of perception of a situation is increased if one is able to identify one's own feelings, attitudes, limitations, capabilities, etc.

(c) Clarity of perception of a situation may require a change in perception or correction of misconceptions.

(d) Clarity of perception of a situation may require an opportunity for experiences in an actual situation in addition to or rather than hearing a verbal description of such a situation.

(e) Clarity of perception of a situation may be increased by verbal exploration of the situation in the presence of an informed and supportive person.

(f) Inconsistency, confusion and multiplicity of demands on the part of others in the environment may contribute to lack of clarity in perception of the situation.

(3) A feeling of comfort and safety in coping with life situations is more likely to be increased if one is able to identify and accept one's own current and potential abilities, limitations, feelings, attitudes, etc.

(4) An individual is more likely to achieve a feeling of comfort and safety in coping with life situations if he has an understanding of action to be taken and possession of the skills and abilities necessary for the action.

(a) Security in life situations is likely to be increased as the individual gains more experience (skill) in coping with the specific situation.

(b) The acquisition of skills necessary for successful action requires the opportunity for adequate learning experiences.

(5) For some individuals, or in some situations, a feeling of comfort and safety requires that the individual maintain control of himself and the situation, regardless of the actual necessity for such control.

(a) Most individuals in our culture will experience

anxiety if deprived of the opportunity or right to make decisions regarding self and personal property.

(b) Frustration of one's efforts toward a specific goal constitute loss of control over the situation.

(c) Dependence upon others imposed by illness constitutes loss of control over a situation.

(d) For some individuals a feeling of comfort and safety is achieved through controlling or manipulating the environment and the people in it.

(6) A feeling of comfort and safety in handling life situations may be achieved by the establishment of familiar routines, behavior patterns and environmental circumstances which have been previously experienced as safe and comfortable.

(a) A feeling of comfort and safety in coping with life situations is enhanced if the individual has had previous similar experiences in which he has not been harmed.

(b) Any interference with or change in normal physiological and/or psychological functioning is likely to cause psychological disequilibrium because: it may be perceived as a threat to life; it may require new, unknown patterns of behavior which have not been experienced as satisfactory; unknown consequences may be feared.

(c) Illness and/or hospitalization disrupts previously established behavior patterns.

(7) A feeling of safety and comfort in a specific situation may be increased by positive preparation before the situation occurs.

(a) Positive preparation for a potentially threatening event may include increasing one's knowledge about the event.

(b) Positive preparation for a potentially threatening event may include changing one's perception of the event.

(c) Positive preparation for a potentially threatening event may include verbalization about the event in the presence of a supportive person.

(d) Positive preparation for a potentially threatening event may include the opportunity for vicarious successful experience through discussion with someone who has lived through the event successfully.

(e) Positive preparation for a potentially threatening event may include an opportunity to learn skills necessary for mastery of the situation.

(8) Disturbances of physiological or psycho-social equilibrium which result in exaggerated emotional reactions or mental dysfunction will decrease the individual's ability to cope successfully with life situations.

(a) Internal and external confusion interferes with an individual's control of his own behavior.

(b) In extremely threatening situations an individual may need constant repetition of successful experiences before tension can be decreased sufficiently to allow the individual to successfully cope with a situation.

(c) A high degree of apprehension may interfere with an individual's ability to successfully cope with a situation.

(d) Clarity, simplicity and lack of threat in the way others approach a confused person facilitates cooperation between the confused person and others in the environment and the feeling of comfort and safety of the confused person.

B. A feeling of comfort and safety in a specific situation may be increased by identification with others who have experienced the situation without harm.

C. Comfort and safety in a situation may be increased by the possession of material objects which symbolically represent safety and comfort.

D. A feeling of comfort and safety may be achieved through relationships with others.

(1) A feeling of comfort and safety may be achieved through dependence upon or cooperation with others.

(a) Cooperation between individuals is dependent upon adequate communication between the individuals involved.

(b) In a situation where the individual must depend upon others, a feeling of safety and comfort depends upon the assurance (knowledge) that help is available for satisfaction of basic needs of one's self and one's dependents.

(c) An individual may be helped to feel safe and comfortable in a dependent situation if he receives a positive interpretation of on-going events.

(d) The achievement of a feeling of comfort and safety through dependence upon or cooperation with others requires that the individual be able to trust and have confidence in others.

Confidence in others is likely to be increased upon the assurance that all matters pertaining to one's self will be considered confidential.

Confidence in others is partially dependent upon the assurance that others are competent to carry out tasks assigned or entrusted to them.

Confidence in others is partially dependent upon the assurance that others have a genuine concern for the health and welfare of the individual who is dependent.

Confidence in others is partially dependent upon the consistency of attitude and behavior of those upon whom one must depend.

In order to trust and have confidence in others, one must have repeated experiences involving people whom one perceives as trustworthy and honest.

The suspicious or doubtful person may be able to cooperate with others if he receives realistic interpretation and encouragement from someone whom he trusts.

The person who is suspicious, doubtful or fearful will react with increased suspicion and fear if other individuals in the environment show doubt and lack of control.

(2) A feeling of comfort and safety may be achieved through the mutual sharing of responsibility with others whom one trusts or for whom one cares.

(a) The inclusion of an individual's family in a situation may increase the feeling of safety and comfort by the sharing of responsibility within the family group.

(b) In a threatening situation, an individual may receive the greatest support from a member of the family or some individual with whom a close affectional bond exists.

(3) A feeling of safety and comfort may be achieved through relationships with others which realistically indicate that the individual will not be harmed or allowed to come to harm.

(a) Psychological support and assistance may be given through the attitudes and behaviors of others in the situation.

The suspicious, doubtful or fearful individual can frequently be helped to feel safe and comfortable in a situation if others in the situation are, or appear to be, calm, self-assured and in control of the situation.

An attitude of objectivity on the part of others in the situation may help the individual to feel safe and comfortable.

In some situations, setting limits or giving firm directions will be helpful in assisting a person to feel safe, comfortable and competent.

A feeling of comfort and safety may be enhanced by the presence of a warm, understanding person.

The realistically based approval and encouragement of others contributes to one's feeling of safety and comfort in a situation.

An individual's feeling of security may be increased by being made to feel welcome in strange or unfamiliar surroundings.

Physical care procedures may be used as a means of giving emotional support and may help in the establishment of positive interpersonal relations.

(b) Actions by others motivated by the anticipation of an individual's needs tends to increase one's feeling of safety and comfort.

(c) If an individual experiences a feeling of acceptance and esteem in relation to other individuals, he will be better able to tolerate criticism, correction or guidance from those individuals with a minimum of discomfort.

(4) A feeling of comfort and safety in life situations requires that the individual experience a feeling of approval and acceptance by others.

(5) For most individuals, a feeling of comfort and safety in life situations requires that the individual experience a feeling of relatedness to others.

E. The ability to communicate one's needs is prerequisite to a feeling of safety and comfort.

F. A feeling of safety and comfort may be achieved through religious beliefs and practices.

G. A feeling of safety and comfort requires the absence of threat to the life and integrity of the organism.

(1) The presence of persons who are in ill health or who are diseased may constitute a threat to the life of other individuals, either through fear of contracting the illness or through the symbolic implications the illness might have.

(2) The presence of hostility in the environment may have implications for potential danger.

(3) Any interference with or change in normal physiological and/or psychological function is usually perceived as a threat to the life or integrity of the organism.

(4) Any use of physical force by one person upon another person may constitute (symbolically or realistically) a threat to the integrity or life of the organism.

(5) Illness/hospitalization realistically or symbolically implies an existing threat to the life and integrity of the organism.

(6) The presence of dead or dying persons in the environment usually produces anxiety in other individuals in the environment.

5. The needs of a specific individual at a given time will vary according to internal and external factors.
   A. The needs of a specific individual at a given time are partially determined by the nature of the organism.
   B. The needs of a specific individual at a given time are partially determined by the individual's membership in a specific socio-cultural group.
   C. The needs of a specific individual at a given time are partially determined by the individual's past living experiences.
   D. The needs of a specific individual at a given time are partially determined by the individual's current life situations.

(1) Illness and/or hospitalization disturbs the individual's pattern of need satisfaction.

(2) Certain needs of the individual are intensified by physical illness.

(3) Certain needs of the individual are more difficult to

satisfy if he is physically ill and/or hospitalized.

(4) Inherent in illness and/or hospitalization are potentially traumatic elements or problem situations to which the individual must make some form of adaptation.

(5) Of the complex of more or less intense needs of a specific individual at a given time, those needs which are most intense take priority over those needs creating less tension.

II

NURSING CARE RELATED TO THE PRINCIPLES AND HYPOTHESES

1. "In order to achieve and maintain psychological equilibrium, man must have satisfying relationships with other human beings, both individually and in groups."

   A. "The feeling of being cared for or about by another person is necessary for psychological homeostasis." The nurse can help the patient to feel cared for by:

   (1) Giving him physical care and assistance with an attitude which indicates that he is important and worthy of her concern.

   (2) Listening attentively to what he has to say and showing an interest in him and his activities.

   (3) Arranging her care plans to include and encourage visits from those who are affectionally close to the patient.

   (4) Demonstrating concern regarding his health and welfare by her inquiries and her attention to details of care.

   (5) Showing consideration for his particular preferences in the nursing care situation.

   (6) Making him feel welcome and cared for by her attitude upon admission and in nurse-patient situations thereafter.

   (7) Giving him special attention if the need in this area is greater than usual.

B. "The awareness that one is not alone is basic to psychological homeostasis." The nurse can help to prevent or alleviate feelings of aloneness by:

(1) Providing for someone to be with the patient when he is undergoing particularly traumatic experiences.

(2) Providing the patient with non-threatening information about other people who have had similar experiences.

(3) Providing time for visiting with friends, relatives, other patients and/or nurses.

(4) Indicating that she understands (empathizes with) him.

(5) Arranging the environment so that he is aware of the presence of others who are concerned with his welfare.

C. "The approval of others in one's socio-cultural environment is necessary for psychological homeostasis." The nurse may provide the patient with experiences in which he feels approval by:

(1) Giving him the opportunity to behave in socially approved ways, especially in situations where his behavior will be noticed by others. (e.g., shaving the male patient or attention to hair and make-up for the female patient.)

(2) Preventing situations which will cause the patient to feel disapproval. (e.g., nursing measures to prevent excessive soiling of the bed for the incontinent patient.)

(3) Maintaining an attitude of respect and consideration while giving care.

(4) Voicing sincere approval of patient behavior whenever his behavior merits approval.

(5) Seeking out opportunities or creating opportunities for voicing approval if the patient need in this area is greater than usual.

(6) Controlling her own behavior to prevent showing of attitudes which indicate disapproval (unless disapproval is therapeutically indicated.)

D. "Acceptance of one's self and one's individual differences by others is necessary for psychological homeostasis." The nurse can assist the patient to feel that he is accepted by:
   (1) Her attitude of understanding and empathy.
   (2) Providing him with opportunities for social interaction with others when this is feasible.
   (3) Her consideration for his preferences or individual differences while giving care.
   (4) Avoiding situations which would cause him to feel unaccepted.
   (5) Control of her behavior to show acceptance in situations where the patient is likely to anticipate non-acceptance. (e.g. disfigurement, malfunction, uncontrollable behavior which is non-harmful.)

E. "In order to experience satisfying relationships with others, the average individual must be able to feel that he will not be harmed as a result of the relationship." The nurse can assist the patient to feel safe in nurse-patient relationships by:
   (1) Her attitude and actions which indicate concern, approval, acceptance or protection.
   (2) Arranging for continuity of care from one person (or as few persons as possible) so that the patient will be able to know those who care for him well enough to be comfortable with them.
   (3) The re-assignment of personnel who do not threaten the patient when it becomes known that a particular staff member is threatening to the patient.
   (4) Being consistent in her attitude and behavior so that the patient can feel comfortable with her.
   (5) Being especially gentle, kind, patient and understanding when the patient indicates that he is unusually fearful in interpersonal situations.
   (6) Demonstrating competence in all areas of nursing care.

F. "The achievement of satisfying relationships with others is influenced by the psycho-physiological structure and function of the organism." The nurse can further assist the patient toward satisfying relationships with others by:

(1) Showing acceptance of his limitations and approval of his abilities.

(2) Helping him to adjust to changes in self-concept when such changes are necessary.

   (a) Providing opportunities for satisfying experiences according to the requirements of the change.

   (b) Acquainting him with facts which have a bearing on his future adjustment.

   (c) Showing acceptance and approval while he is undergoing new experiences and/or adjusting to a new role.

(3) Assisting him in establishing adequate communications.

   (a) Using terminology or other communicative symbols which he will understand.

   (b) Helping him to learn additional means for communication when necessary.

   (c) Helping to clarify the communications of others.

(4) Teaching him health care practices which will prevent disapproval or non-acceptance from others, especially when his physical condition is conducive to such attitudes. (i.e. colostomy care, use of prosthetic equipment.)

(5) Helping him toward self-acceptance and greater self-esteem by her attitude of acceptance and approval.

(6) Encouraging him to express and explore his feelings about others without showing judgment of his feelings.

(7) Providing understanding support and/or encouragement while he explores his relationships with others and makes decisions regarding changes in existing relationships.

G. "The achievement of satisfying relationships with others is influenced by socio-cultural factors." The nurse can further assist the patient toward satisfying relationships with others by:

(1) Helping him to clarify his perception of the socio-cultural role of himself and others.
(2) Helping him to learn socio-culturally approved forms of behavior.
(3) Assisting him to examine his own behavior and how it may effect others.
(4) Providing him with knowledge and positive experiences in relation to other individuals who have ideas, attitudes and/or forms of behavior different from his own.
(5) Preventing his being placed in interpersonal situations which will cause stress. (i.e. male patient being assisted with elimination process by female nurse; placing a minority group in a room with a person who is prejudiced against that group.)
(6) Assisting him to carry out actions required by the particular socio-cultural group to which he belongs. (i.e. diet requirements for some religious groups; etc.)
(7) Her attitude of acceptance regarding patient behavior required by the particular socio-cultural group to which the patient belongs.

2. "The achievement and maintenance of psychological equilibrium is enhanced if the individual has a sense of self-esteem." This statement has implications for nursing care in the following ways:
   A. The nurse can assist the patient in maintaining satisfying relationships with others.
   B. The nurse can help the patient to feel useful and needed by:
      (1) Asking for his opinion and preference whenever possible in nursing care situations.
      (2) Asking for or encouraging the patient to assist with his own care whenever possible or feasible.
      (3) Arranging for the patient to assist in carrying out tasks and procedures in the hospital if the patient's need in this area is greater than usual. (i.e. delivering

mail, writing for other patients, copying cards for Kardex, etc.)

(4) Encouraging the patient's friends and family to do things which will maintain or increase his feeling of being needed and useful.

C. The nurse can help the patient to maintain his sense of self-esteem by the control of her attitude and behavior in nurse-patient situations by:

(1) Showing respect and consideration in all nurse-patient situations.

(2) Avoiding any negative attitudes (dislike, ridicule, indifference, hostility) which might cause the patient to suffer decreased self-esteem.

D. The nurse can help the patient to maintain his sense of self-esteem by assisting him to live in accordance with socio-cultural standards, especially those which he sees valuable. She can do this by:

(1) Encouraging or allowing him to be self-directing.

(2) Recognizing and respecting his individual differences.

(3) Showing respect for the socio-cultural group to which the patient belongs.

(4) Helping the patient to act in accordance with the requirements of the socio-cultural group to which he may belong. (i.e. dietary or other religious practices.)

(5) Avoiding embarrassing situations which could result from physiological inability to live or behave in accordance with socially approved standards of behavior.

(a) Physical care procedures to minimize embarrassment due to incontinence, body odor due to disease processes, inability to feed self, etc.

(b) Matter-of-fact and accepting attitude when giving care which might cause embarrassment.

(6) Helping the patient to change his concept of a situation and to accept his own disabilities when he is physically or mentally unable to live according to previously acquired standards:

(a) By her attitude of approval and acceptance.
(b) By supplying information which the patient might not have regarding his change in status.
(c) By providing compensatory experiences to make up for deficiencies.
(d) By interpreting situations to family and friends.
(e) See principles Section IV for other socially approved behaviors.

3. "In order to achieve and maintain psychological equilibrium, the individual must have an adequate means of self-definition and situational definition." The nurse can assist the patient in this area by:
   A. Demonstrating, through attitude and behavior, her recognition of the patient's individuality. (i.e. calling him by name; recalling—and referring to in discussions—information about the patient's life and background such as hobby and home interests, children, work.)
   B. Assisting the patient to acquire necessary information about the situation he is in. The nurse can assist the patient by:
      (1) Orienting him to new situations.
      (2) Explaining or providing information about activities in the environment, especially those in which he might become involved. (i.e. doctor's rounds, call systems, etc.)
      (3) Providing information (or seeing that it is provided by appropriate people) about his illness and treatment.
   C. Assisting the patient to maintain self and situational orientation when he has some perceptual handicap. The nurse can assist the patient by:
      (1) Constant use of his name when he is confused.
      (2) Constant referral or drawing of attention to surroundings to provide re-orientation when the patient is confused or has a very short memory or attention span.
      (3) Assignment of the patient to a minimum number of nursing personnel to avoid further confusion when

the patient is confused or has a defective memory.

(4) Repetition of information which the patient might need for orientation (i.e. referring to the doctor's name, referring to time and circumstances regarding care and treatment).

D. Allowing or encouraging the patient to utilize convictions and beliefs for orientation. The nurse can assist the patient in this area by:

(1) Arranging for visits from minister or priest.

(2) Procuring material objects or providing for practices which the patient might use for self and situational orientation. (i.e. Bible, communion, etc.)

(3) Allowing or encouraging the patient to talk about convictions and beliefs which are reassuring, and strengthening these beliefs if feasible.

E. Providing for or encouraging the patient's identification with or sharing of experiences with others. This implies:

(1) Referring, in discussion, to others who have similar characteristics, needs, etc.

(2) Providing information about other individuals who have similar characteristics, needs, etc. through writing, reading.

F. Helping the patient to identify and learn to behave in accordance with his role in relation to others. This implies:

(1) Orienting the patient to the hospital social structure and his place in the structure.

(2) Orientation of the patient to possible changes in his role and status which might be necessitated by the nature of his illness.

(3) Providing encouragement and support as the patient learns how to behave in accordance with changed self-concept. (Avoiding criticism, gently correcting inappropriate behavior, giving approval for adequate behavior.)

(4) Correcting misconceptions regarding appropriate role and behavior in situations with which he is unfamiliar.

G. Providing for or allowing the maintenance or establishment of familiar and consistent routines and behavior patterns which the patient might use for self and situational orientation. This implies:
   (1) Allowing or encouraging the patient to have and to use personal objects from his home environment. (i.e. pajamas or other clothing from home, personal toilet articles, other articles of significance to the patient, such as blanket or pillow.)
   (2) Allowing or encouraging personal care or activity routines which the patient may have established at home. (i.e. individual habits, recreational or occupational activities.)
   (3) Encouraging or allowing visits from friends and relatives.
   (4) Assignment of as few nursing personnel as possible, and consistent assignment of those personnel, to allow for establishment of familiar patterns of care by familiar people.
   (5) Setting up of consistent routines of care in the hospital by which the patient may orient himself.
   (6) Prevention of disruption of individual routines and behavior patterns whenever possible.
   (7) Demonstrating consistency of attitude and behavior herself.

H. Whenever a change in self or situational orientation is necessitated by illness or hospitalization, providing support and encouragement until a new means of orientation has been established. This implies:
   (1) See other behaviors in this section, plus:
   (2) Providing for extra attention or attendance when the patient may be apprehensive.
   (3) Giving constant approval for new desired behaviors.
   (4) Pointing out realistic advantages of changed self or situational conditions.

I. Avoiding behaviors or situations which tend to cause disorientation. This implies:

(1) Minimizing confusion in the environment.
(2) Avoiding sudden changes, especially without sufficient situational definition.
(3) Avoiding demands on the patient for which he has not been prepared.

4. "In order to establish and maintain psychological equilibrium, the individual will attempt to achieve a feeling of safety and comfort in life situations." The nurse can help the patient in this area by:

A. Assisting and encouraging the patient to cope with situations with success and satisfaction. This implies:
(1) Providing him with necessary information about the situation.
(2) Correcting any misconceptions he may have about the situations.
(3) Providing opportunity for perceptional experiences which will familiarize him with the situation.
(4) Assisting him to define the actions he can and should take.
(5) Assisting him to take the actions necessary.
(6) Allowing or encouraging him to discuss the situation in order to clarify his own thinking.
(7) Making sure that directions are clearly given and within the patient's ability to understand.
(8) Helping him to clarify or understand his role in a situation.
(9) Assisting him in the definition and acceptance of his own abilities, limitations, feelings, etc., in the situation. (i.e. asking thought-provoking questions, pointing out possibilities, giving encouragement and approval.)
(10) Providing the patient with opportunities to learn new skills and habits required for successful action in a situation. (Implies the use of principles of learning.)
(11) Allowing the patient to retain control of himself and the situation insofar as possible. (i.e. asking

his opinion or preference, letting him plan or help to plan care which concerns him, avoiding actions which remove control from his jurisdiction.)

(12) Avoiding actions which will result in frustration of the patient's aims and goals whenever possible.

(13) Providing necessary correction, guidance or limitations with an attitude of gentleness and concern for the patient's welfare.

(14) Providing additional safe opportunities for the patient to experience a feeling of control if he demonstrates excessive needs in this area.

(15) Providing for or allowing the maintenance and establishment of routines and consistent patterns of behavior in which the patient has the opportunity to feel safe and comfortable.

(16) Pointing out or helping the patient to see relationships between familiar (past) routines and activities and new situations.

(17) Giving the patient emotional support and encouragement when he is faced with disruption in familiar patterns and behavior.

(18) Using the patient's previously acquired knowledge and skill in the adaptation to new situations whenever possible.

(19) Avoiding disruption of familiar routines whenever possible.

(20) Providing for adequate preparation for expected events. In addition to specific actions stated in other sections, this implies:

(a) Seeing that the patient is physically comfortable.

(b) Providing for assistance, or letting the patient know that assistance will be available.

(c) Attempting to remove or relieve additional fears and worries the patient might have in order to leave him free to concentrate on the new experience without distraction.

(21) Removing, eliminating or decreasing factors which interfere with the patient's successful action in a situation. This implies:
   (a) Avoiding confusion.
   (b) Avoiding distraction.
   (c) Providing for clarity and simplicity if the patient is already confused.
   (d) Providing constant repetition of direction and guidance if the patient is confused or emotionally disturbed.
   (e) Decreasing fear or worry whenever possible.

(22) Providing necessary equipment.

B. Assisting the patient to identify with others who have achieved safety and success in similar situations.

C. Providing for or allowing the patient to have possession of and use material objects which, for him, symbolize safety and comfort. (i.e. objects from home; objects that he may request; objects the nurse can provide.)

D. Demonstrating through her attitude and behavior, or arranging for the presence of others whose attitude and behavior will demonstrate that the patient will be safe and comfortable. This implies:
   (1) Demonstrating competence and capability in nurse-patient situations.
   (2) Anticipation of and attempts to satisfy patient needs and desires before the patient makes requests.
   (3) Demonstrating an attitude of concern for the patient's welfare.
   (4) Providing safe guidance with an attitude of kindness and concern.
   (5) Demonstration of understanding and acceptance of the individual patient and his needs, actions, desires, etc.
   (6) Making known to the patient sources of assistance and information.
   (7) Assisting the patient to communicate needs, desires, feelings.

(8) Interpreting or providing information about current events or situations.
(9) Behaving in such a way as to foster the patient's trust and confidence.
(10) Encouraging or allowing the patient to share experiences with those who are affectionally close. (i.e. including family members in care plans and teaching of care procedure; allowing family or friends to visit, especially when patient is undergoing traumatic experiences; helping family to understand and support the patient.)
(11) Demonstration, consistently, of attitudes of understanding, acceptance, approval, interest, concern, non-judgment.
(12) Providing for the physical presence of a supportive person when the patient is involved in frightening experiences.

E. Assisting the patient to communicate his needs, desires, feelings, etc.

F. Allowing or encouraging religious practices through which the patient may achieve a feeling of safety and comfort.

G. Removing, decreasing or avoiding situations or actions which might constitute a threat to the life or integrity of the individual person. This implies:
(1) Management of the environment to avoid contact with patients who have communicable disease, frightening symptoms, or symptoms from which the patient might draw implications for himself.
(2) Management of the environment to avoid situations which would allow the patient to see dead or dying persons, or hear them discussed.
(3) Management of the environment to avoid overhearing staff discussion of other patients or himself.
(4) Control of her own (and others') attitude and behavior to avoid demonstration of hostility and aggression, either between patients, between patient and staff or between staff members.
(5) Avoidance of changes in behavior and practices

which were perceived as safe whenever possible.

(6) Avoiding the use of physical force or the suggestions, real or symbolic, of force whenever possible. This implies:
   (a) Providing for someone to be with the patient rather than using mechanical restraints.
   (b) Providing an attitude of kindness and concern, with adequate orientation and re-orientation as to the reasons for such restraint, when mechanical restraints are necessary.
   (c) Utilizing medication orders and nursing care measures to avoid use of mechanical restraints.

(7) Utilizing all opportunities to accentuate the positive aspects of hospitalization and health care. (i.e. planning for future return to optimum health, avoiding traumatic experiences, preparation for health care procedures, etc.)

(8) Providing for physical safety and comfort in the environment. (See Natural Sciences.)

5. "The needs of a specific individual at a given time will vary according to internal and external factors." The nurse can assist the patient in this area by:
   A. Acquainting herself with facts about the individual patient.
   B. Acquainting herself with facts about the requirements of the patient's particular socio-cultural group.
   C. Acquainting herself with facts about the patient's past experiences, especially as they pertain to current events in the patient's life situation.
   D. Attempting to determine the patient's most immediate needs and those which are pressing, but secondary.

SECTION D

Social Science Principles and Hypotheses and Related Nursing Care for the Concepts:

"Social and cultural institutions exist as a result of the needs of man (individually and collectively) and must be maintained for the preservation of man's psycho-social and psycho-biological equilibrium."

and

"The individual tends to seek satisfaction of his needs within his culture and through the channels which that culture has established for satisfaction of individual needs."

I

SOCIAL SCIENCE PRINCIPLES AND HYPOTHESES

1. The society or culture in which an individual lives helps to determine the ways in which his needs are met.
   A. A specific culture may provide alternative ways of satisfying a specific human need.
   B. Social agencies are formed as a result of unsatisfied needs of the individual and/or groups of individuals in the society.
   C. In the process of growth and development, many cultural values become internalized to the point where they are no longer seen as socio-cultural requirements but are experienced as subjective ideas, attitudes, beliefs, needs, etc. of the individual.
2. Acceptance by society requires that the individual behave in a manner prescribed by the society of which he is a member.
   A. Socially acceptable adjustment requires that the indi-

vidual learn acceptable methods for expressions of emotions, thoughts, feelings, etc.

B. Any given activity may be considered normal or healthy in one situation and abnormal or unhealthy in another situation, dependent upon cultural definition.

C. In every society or culture, there are established rules and codes of conduct governing the relationships of members of the opposite sex and members of the same sex.
   (1) In our culture, physical exposure in the presence of a member of the opposite sex is governed by specific rules and codes.

   No additional statements emerged from the data.

D. Every society or culture provides means for establishing and ascribing roles of authority, subordinate and peer positions, and the behavior appropriate to each role and the relationships between role assignees.
   (1) In our own culture, doctors are usually seen in a role of authority.
   (2) In our society, authority figures are regarded with respect, awe and, frequently, fear.

E. Societies which have more than one racial or religious group will have some systematized codes for behavior regarding the role, status, intergroup relations, etc., between these groups.
   (1) In a society where there are multiple racial and religious groups, satisfactory interpersonal relationships may be interfered with because of preconceived ideas, misconceptions, and lack of knowledge regarding socially approved behavioral limits.
   (2) Individuals who belong to minority or fringe groups within a society usually experience some feeling of insecurity or inadequacy by reason of belonging to a group which is not accepted as a part of the majority group.

F. Every society or culture has established rules and codes of conduct governing the roles and relationships of family members.

(1) In our society, certain types of parental rejection of children are frowned upon.

No additional statements emerged from the data.

G. In every society or culture, there are established rules and codes of conduct governing voluntary physiological functions and physical appearance.

(1) In our culture, the control of eliminative processes and associated procedures is governed by comparatively rigid standards.

(2) In our culture, physical cleanliness and the appearance of neatness are socially approved (desired) attributes.

H. In every society or culture there are established customs and beliefs governing attitudes and behaviors regarding illness and death.

(1) In some cultures, attendance at the bedside of a dying person by specified other individuals is socially approved.

(2) In every culture, there are some physical conditions or diseases which have negative connotations.

I. Every society or culture places positive or negative value on certain general attitudes, ideas, beliefs and their attendant actions and gives or withholds approval of the individual according to his conformance to these standards.

(1) In our culture, personal adequacy, independence and self-control are highly valued attributes.

(a) In our culture, self-direction and independent action are considered basic human rights.

(b) In our culture, any action which is perceived by the individual as a threat to independence or freedom (right to select action by free choice) is most likely to be resisted.

(2) In our society, respect and consideration are considered basic human rights.

(3) In some groups, personal privacy is highly valued.

(4) In some societies and in some situations, the suppression of overt hostility is required.

(5) In some cultures, individual possession, ownership and subsequent disposal of material objects has significance and is governed by customs and laws set up by that culture.

J. Some socio-cultural and/or personal values, attitudes, beliefs, etc., which originally arose from a basic need have attained a significance sufficient to guide behavior, even though the original need for the attitude, belief, behavior, etc., no longer exists.

K. Knowledge of social role is learned through contact with the social environment in which the individual has the opportunity to see and practice the designated role.

3. A basic factor in the continued existence of a group is that the interaction of group members continues to satisfy the desires and needs of its members.

A. Effective communication is prerequisite to effective social interaction.

B. Groups of people can work effectively toward a common goal if communication between members of the group is adequate.

C. Occasionally problem situations in interpersonal situations can be solved by removing one or more individuals from the group.

D. Socio-cultural groups facilitate ease in interpersonal relations by establishing certain cultural patterns, forms of behavior and common activities.

(1) Social conventions facilitate effective interpersonal relations by making clear what is expected of the individuals engaged in those relationships.

(2) In the development of any large group, there occurs a differentiation of the social roles of the individual members of the group.

E. Cooperation and effective group action are facilitated if the individuals involved have a feeling of mutual trust.

F. Efforts to reach a given goal are more likely to be stimulated if the people involved feel that their efforts are appreciated or that they are contributing something of value.

G. The feelings, attitudes and actions of each person in a situation modify the feelings, attitudes and actions of other persons in the same situation.

II

NURSING CARE RELATED TO THE PRINCIPLES AND HYPOTHESES

1. "The society or culture in which an individual lives helps to determine the ways in which his needs are met." "Acceptance by society requires that the individual behave in a manner prescribed by the society of which he is a member." The nurse can broaden her awareness of socio-cultural forces in the individual patient's life in order to:
   A. Assist the patient to behave in accordance with the requirements of his particular socio-cultural group when this is necessary to the patient's emotional security.
   B. Maintain an attitude of acceptance and understanding regarding the patient's behavior (socio-culturally derived) when it may deviate from her own expected standards.
   C. Inform the patient, as necessary, regarding social agencies which may assist him in the satisfaction of his needs.
   D. Assist the patient to increase his awareness of socio-culturally approved behaviors in order to decrease his apprehension of others, increase his understanding and acceptance of others and increase his potential range of acceptable behavior.
   E. Avoid criticism, ridicule, embarrassment or other discomforts for the patient as a result of violation of any of his culturally derived standards or values.
   F. Control her own behavior in accordance with socially approved standards whenever necessary for therapeutic benefit of the patient.
   G. Increase her own understanding of how her behavior may be influenced by socio-cultural standards.
   H. Assist the patient to change his self-expectations and expectations of others (as based on socio-cultural standards) when necessitated by the patient's physiological or psychological status.

2. "A basic factor in the continued existence of a group is that the interaction of group members continues to satisfy the desires and needs of its members." The nurse can utilize knowledge in this area to increase her effectiveness as a member of the health team by:
   A. Assisting in the maintenance of effective communications between herself and other health team members and between the patient and the health team.
   B. Assisting in the definition of goals to be reached by the health team and keeping herself informed as to the goals of the health team.
   C. Helping the patient to keep informed as to the goals of the health care program.
   D. Assisting in the interpretation of the patient's goals to other members of the health team.
   E. Increasing her awareness of and ability to operate in accordance with the requirements of her assigned role in the health team.
   F. Assisting other members of the health team in understanding and acting in accord with assigned roles.
   G. Interpreting to the patient the role and function of health team members with whom he may come in contact.
   H. Promoting effective group relations through an application of principles of human behavior.

SECTION E

General Principles of Nursing Care Derived Directly from the Analysis of Data

1. Establishment of a therapeutic environment or therapeutic relationship requires that the health team member be able to identify and act according to the requirements of the professional role in relation to the patient and to other members of the health team.
   A. To achieve maximum therapeutic benefit, health team members must act within a professional role which precludes personal involvement in the patient's problems, manipulative schemes, etc.
   B. The establishment of a therapeutic environment requires that health team members maintain a calm, objective attitude in relation to the patient and his behavior. This may be achieved by, for example:
      (1) Refraining from making value judgments regarding patient behavior, experiences, emotions, conditions, etc.
      (2) Assuming an unprejudiced position until the patient's attitude and/or reasons for action are fully determined.
2. Establishment of a therapeutic environment or therapeutic relationship requires that the health team member be able to examine, evaluate, and control her own behavior in the team member-patient relationship.
   A. Members of the health team may interfere with the therapeutic progress of the patient if their behavior is motivated by personal needs which conflict with the health needs of the patient.

B. Members of the health team may interfere with the therapeutic progress of the patient if they are unaware of their own feelings regarding the patient and are unconsciously reacting to these feelings in patient-staff relations.

C. Emotional demands made upon the patient by health team members are likely to interfere with the therapeutic progress of the patient.

D. The feelings, attitudes, physiological and/or psychological condition of health team members affect patient care through their influence on the behavior of the health team member in staff-patient situations.

E. An understanding of the motivation for a specific behavior may help in decreasing any negative feelings one may have toward the individual exhibiting the behavior.

F. Knowledge and acceptance of one's own current and potential abilities and limitations tends to improve one's ability to function adequately in a situation.

3. Establishment of a therapeutic environment or therapeutic relationship requires the cooperation of health team members and of health team members and patients.

   A. Dissention between health team members (when known to patients) may force the patient to "take sides" and thus decrease his cooperative efforts in the health program.

   B. Dissention between health team members (when known to patients) may cause tension or anxiety for the patient.

   C. Establishment of a therapeutic environment usually requires that patient-staff, patient-patient and staff-staff relations be of a mutually satisfactory nature.

4. Establishment of a therapeutic environment or therapeutic relationship requires that the health team member be able to provide the patient with emotional support in traumatic situations or take action to reduce tension when tension interferes with therapeutic progress.

5. Establishment of a therapeutic environment or therapeutic relationship requires that the health team member be able to establish positive interpersonal relations with the patient.

   A. Establishment of positive interpersonal relations is facilitated if the individuals involved share some experience, knowledge, etc., in common.

B. Positive interpersonal relations are facilitated if the individuals involved experience a feeling of increased self-esteem or acceptance in the relationship.

C. Effective interpersonal relations depend upon the individual's ability to assume the role of another.

D. A feeling of security and self-worth is essential to comfort and satisfaction in interpersonal relations with individuals or groups of individuals.

E. Social conventions facilitate effective interpersonal relationships by making clear what is expected of the individuals involved.

F. An individual's effectiveness in interpersonal relations is increased in direct proportion to his ability to empathize with other individuals in the situation.

G. An individual's attitudes and beliefs influence his behavior in group situations or interpersonal stuations.

6. To be most effective, any therapeutic program must be consistent.